THE PET
FIRST-AID
BOOK

D1681070

HEALTH AND EMERGENCY INFORMATION CARD

1. PET'S NAME _____

2. PET'S BIRTH DATE _____

3. VETERINARIAN: DR. _____

4. PHONE # _____

5. EMERGENCY # _____

6. VACCINATION DATE _____

7. POISON CONTROL CENTER # _____

8. RABIES TAG # _____

9. GROOMER # _____

10. PET-SUPPLY STORE # _____

11. HUMANE SOCIETY # _____

12. NOTES _____

_____

_____

_____

_____

_____

THE PET FIRST-AID BOOK

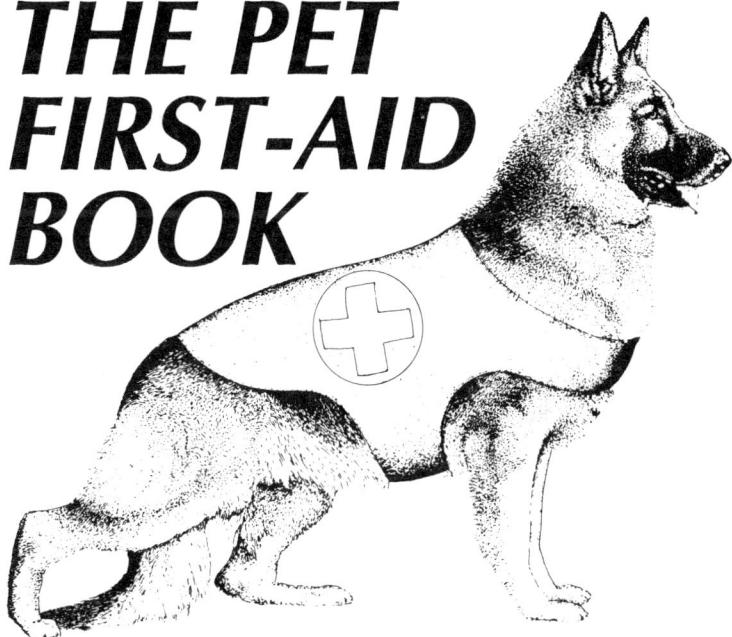

**Dan Hill, D.V.M. / Ann Morrison, D.V.M.
Bernard Myers, D.V.M. / Glenn Finnell, D.V.M.
Genye Hawkins, D.V.M. / Robert Hess, D.V.M.**

of Dan Hill Products, Inc.
Products by Veterinarians ™

McGraw-Hill Book Company

New York St. Louis San Francisco Auckland Bogotá Guatemala
Hamburg Johannesburg Lisbon London Madrid Mexico
Montreal New Delhi Panama Paris San Juan São Paulo
Singapore Sydney Tokyo Toronto

Edited by Ann E. Morrison, D.V.M.
Illustrations and Technical Assistance by Parry Dolle and Mark Pemberton.
Photographs by Rob Alexander and Parry Dolle.

1 2 3 4 5 6 7 8 9 SEMSEM 8 7 6

ISBN 0-07-028892-5

LIBRARY OF CONGRESS CATALOGING-IN-PUBLICATION DATA

Main entry under title:
The Pet first-aid book.
    1. Pets—Diseases.   2. First aid for animals.
I. Hill, Dan, D.V.M.   II. Morrison, Ann, D.V.M.
[DNLM: 1. First Aid—veterinary.   2. Veterinary Medicine
—popular works. SF 751 P477]
SF981.P46   1986   636.089'60252   85-23952
ISBN 0-07-028892-5

Book design by Sharen DuGoff Egana.

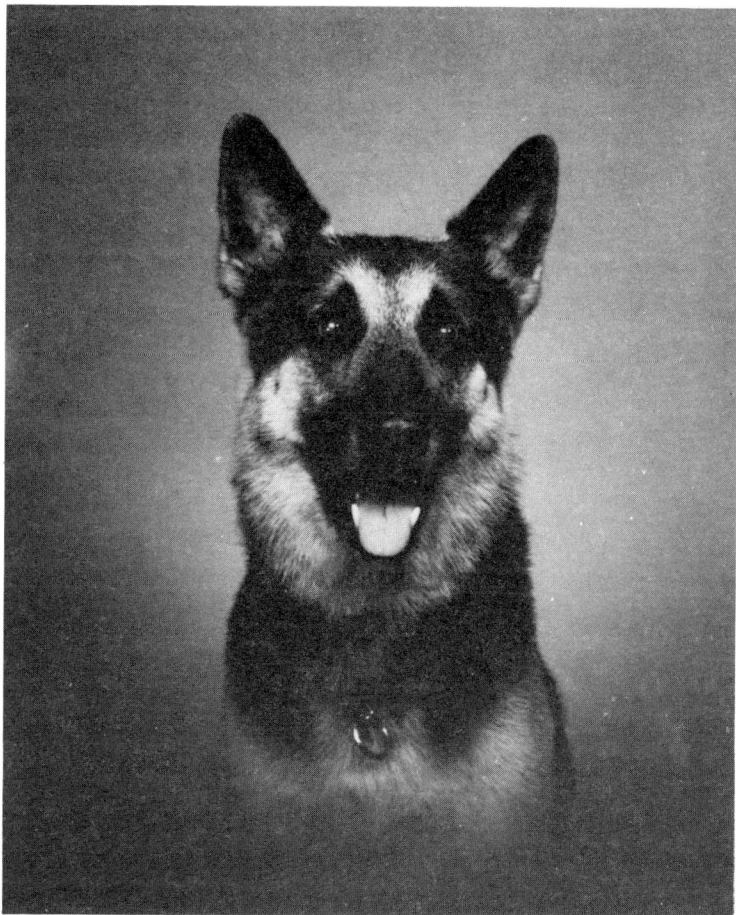

This book is dedicated to the memory of "Duke" Easterling, a police dog with the canine unit of the Orlando, Florida, Police Department. Duke served faithfully and courageously for many years and is credited with three times saving his master's life in the line of duty, the highest service a dog can perform. During his brief retirement with the family of a fellow officer, Duke became a trusted and loyal companion, loved by all.

Duke died October 15, 1984, less than one year after retirement. He epitomized the best, the heart and soul of the dog. Duke will always be loved and missed by those who knew him.

*For people who love and care
for pets and companion animals.*

CONTENTS

CHAPTER THREE
Practicing First Aid   47

x Contents

PREFACE

This book is designed to help you act swiftly and safely in an emergency. It may save your pet's life. It can also teach you many important facts concerning your pet's general health and well-being. We hope the design of the book will make the information easily and almost instantly accessible. Individual chapters will deal with specific aspects of health care, while cross-references will alert you to additional information found elsewhere in the book.

Our introductory chapter, "Practicing Preventive Health Care," sets forth some basic principles which, if followed, may save you many anxious moments later. The second chapter, "Dealing with Common Injuries and Disorders," is the very heart of the book. It presents in synopsis form the symptoms and treatment of health problems common to small pets. Chapter 3, "Practicing First Aid," lays out the techniques often employed in giving emergency treatment to pets. Chapter 4, "Neutering, Breeding, and Birthing," uses charts and photos to enhance your understanding of the reproductive processes of pets.

The final four chapters of this book are devoted to specific discussions of the general care and diet of small domestic animals—birds, caged pets, cats, and dogs—and of the small wild animals that may from time to time fall under your care. The book concludes with an appendix that provides useful miscellaneous information, often bandied about, but collected here for easy reference.

We hope you will find *The Pet First-Aid Book* a ready reference in time of crisis, so that the love you have for your pet can be channeled into helping him or her when help is needed most. Remember, though, that many of these emergencies are serious enough to require the immediate help of a professional.

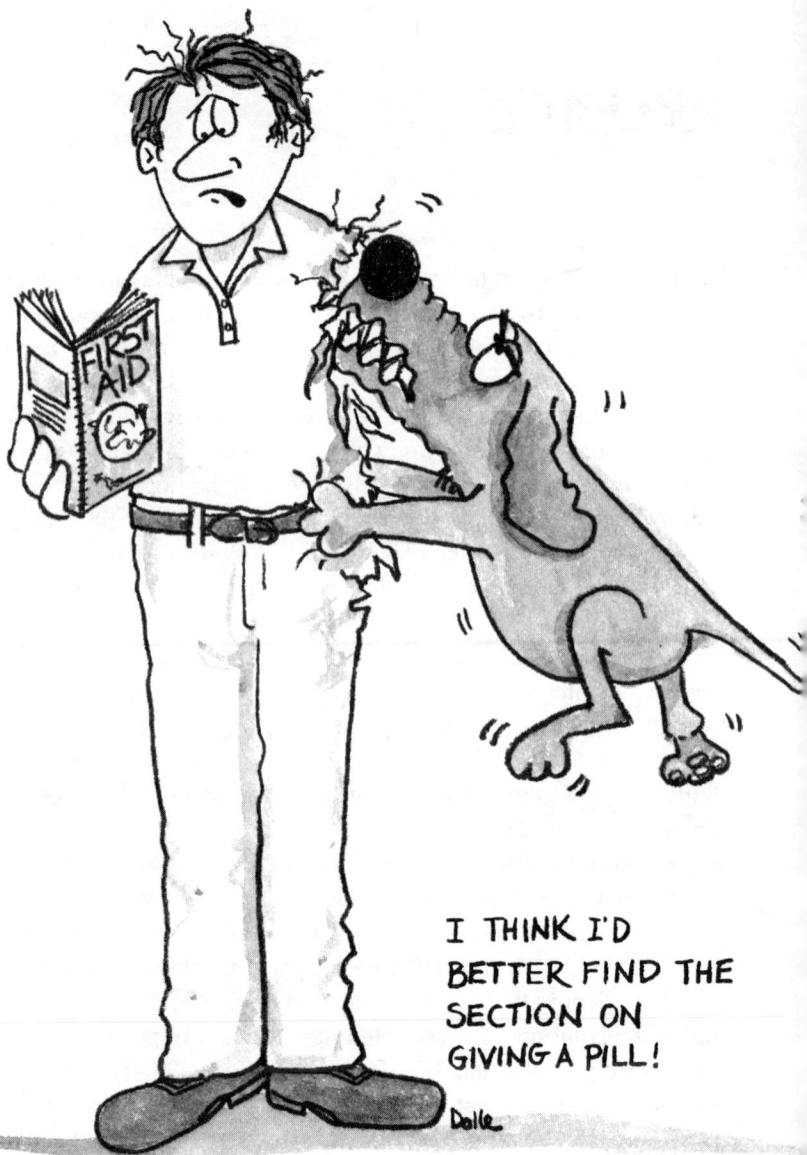

I THINK I'D BETTER FIND THE SECTION ON GIVING A PILL!

CHAPTER ONE

PRACTICING PREVENTIVE HEALTH CARE

The proper care of your pet begins with providing him or her with the environment and diet that are essential to a happy, healthy life. Preventing a problem is always preferable to treating an existing one and is less costly, not only for you but also for your pet.

In order to enjoy your pet for as many years as possible, it is important to discover from your veterinarian exactly what you need to do to keep the animal healthy. Periodic physical examinations will be necessary; prescribed treatment might also include vaccinations, worm checks, heartworm prevention, flea control, and dietary supplements.

Depending on your pet's breed, age, and health condition, there may be special considerations or problems that you need to be made aware of. Ask questions of your veterinarian; no question should be considered too simple or too unimportant where your pet's health is concerned. Establish a good working relationship with your veterinarian and with your pet-supply store.

Subsequent chapters will provide tips for the environment and diet best suited to your specific kind of pet (see Chapters 5, 6, and 7); the following list should serve as a general introductory guide to the basics of preventive health care.

Do ...
Choose the proper size pet to fit your lifestyle and home.
Take your pet to the veterinarian for a physical exam and vaccination.
Feed a high-quality food to your pet.

Keep your pet safely confined at home unless you are walking him on a leash.

Exercise your pet daily.

Leave your pet with plenty of fresh water and shade.

Brush your pet's teeth one to two times weekly.

Help control the pet population by spaying or neutering your animal.

Keep all medications away from pets.

Practice good parasite control for the sake of your pet's health and your own.

Provide your bird with a warm, loving, social environment.

Keep your bird protected and secure from other animals.

Spay or neuter your ferret, unless you intend it to breed.

Use gloves or protective covering when handling ill or stray animals.

Don't . . .

Leave a choke collar on an unattended pet.

Feed your pet prior to a car ride.

Leave your pet in a hot or partially closed car.

Chain your dog where the animal can hang itself.

Put your dog on heartworm prevention until you have him checked by a veterinarian.

Feed real bones to your dog unless your veterinarian recommends them.

Feed dog food to a cat.

Give cats aspirin or aspirin substitutes.

Use lindane (pesticides) or phenol (antiseptics) products on cats.

Leave the dryer or oven door open if you have a cat; they like small spaces.

Leave sewing needles or thread where your cat can get to them.

Use lead paints or lead objects in or around bird cages.

Chain a bird to a perch.

Keep a bird in the kitchen, where some fumes (such as from overheated teflon pans) are hazardous.

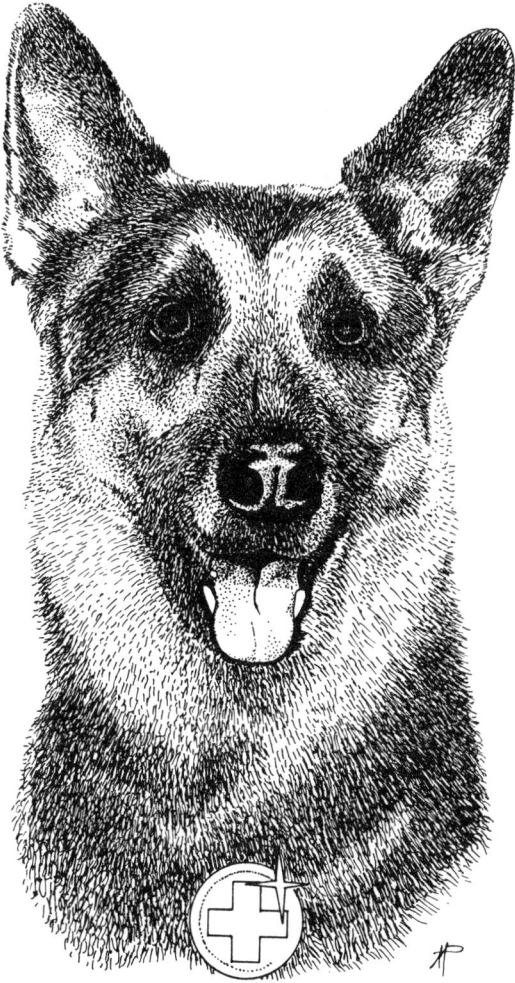

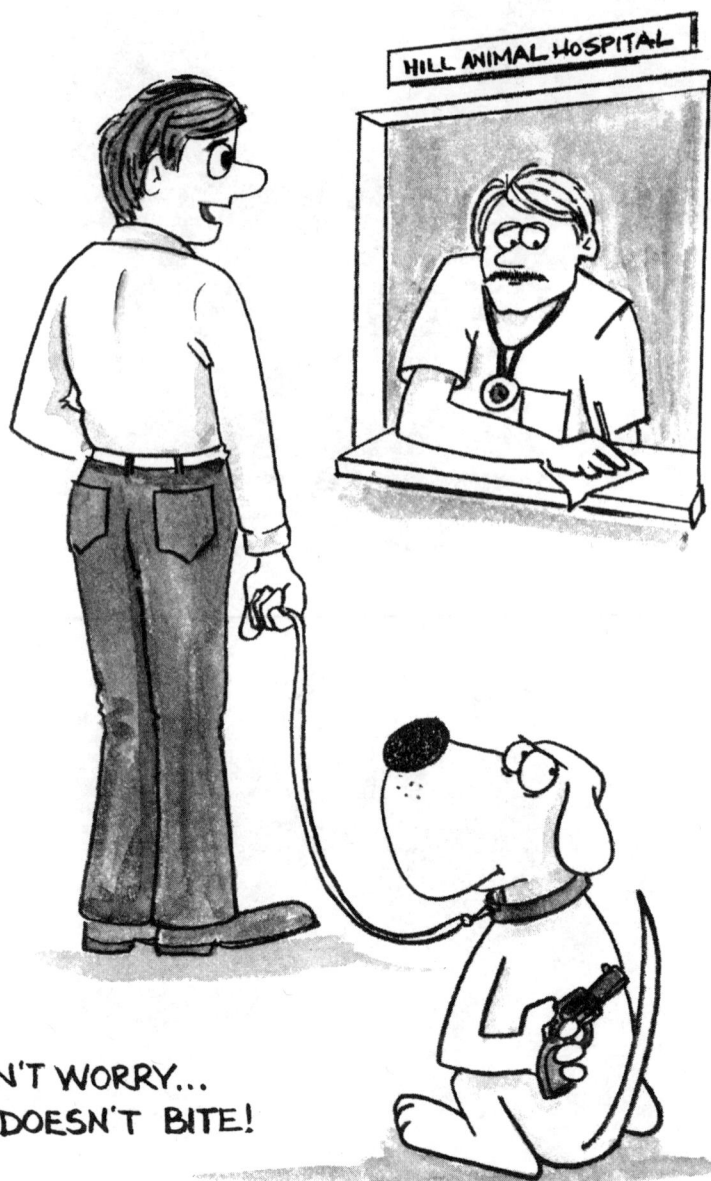

HILL ANIMAL HOSPITAL

DON'T WORRY...
HE DOESN'T BITE!

CHAPTER TWO

DEALING WITH COMMON INJURIES AND DISORDERS

ACCIDENTS

If your pet is involved in any kind of accident, the injuries may cause pain and he may bite. For this reason, muzzling your pet (see How to Muzzle Your Pet, Chapter 3) is a good idea before moving or examining him. Shock and internal injuries are a possibility and a very serious threat to your pet's life. Your veterinarian should always be consulted when there has been an injury.

Treatment:

1. Be sure your pet is breathing. If he is not, gently pull out his tongue, clear his mouth of excessive mucus and debris, and administer artificial respiration by closing his mouth and blowing through his nostrils (see How to Give Artificial Respiration, Chapter 3).
2. Stop any bleeding by applying direct pressure to the area until the bleeding stops, or until it slows enough to enable you to bandage the wound (see How to Stop Bleeding, Chapter 3).
3. Gently splint any injured or broken limb by tying or taping newspapers or a magazine around it (see How to Apply a Splint, Chapter 3). Do this only if it does not cause excessive pain to your pet.
4. Transport your pet to the veterinarian as soon as possible. Avoid unnecessary movement; use a board or other rigid object to load your pet into the car.

Subsequent Care:

In the hours and days that follow an injury, watch for

1. Increasing depression
2. Increasing paleness of the gums
3. A lack of, or decrease in, appetite
4. Problems urinating (which might indicate a ruptured bladder or torn urethra)
5. Continued lameness

If any of these signs occur, see your veterinarian again for further evaluation.

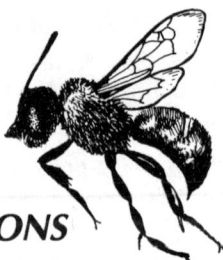

ALLERGIC REACTIONS

Your pet may have a sudden allergic reaction to many things in his or her environment, including insect bites, foods, and drugs.

SEVERE REACTIONS

Severe allergic reactions include (1) restlessness, (2) difficulty in breathing, (3) vomiting or diarrhea, and (4) collapse and/or seizure. In the event of a severe allergic reaction, you must transport your pet to your veterinarian or to the nearest emergency clinic immediately.

MILD REACTIONS

Mild reactions typically include (1) swelling or puffiness around the eyes, mouth, and head; (2) hives on the back and extremities; and (3) itching. In the event of a mild reaction, you can

1. Bathe your pet in cool water for five minutes.
2. Apply a first-aid cream to the irritated skin.
3. See your veterinarian if the condition persists or worsens.

BLEEDING

WARNING: Bleeding from the nose, mouth, or rectum or blood in the urine can be a sign of a severe internal disease, poisoning, or injury. Call your veterinarian immediately.

Severe or prolonged bleeding of any kind can be life-threatening. It is important to act swiftly.

Treatment:
1. Identify the exact area of bleeding.
2. Apply direct pressure to the wound for five minutes with sterile gauze or a clean cloth (see How to Stop Bleeding, Chapter 3). If this is painful to your pet, muzzle him or have someone hold him (see How to Muzzle Your Pet, Chapter 3). If the bleeding does not stop under direct pressure, take your pet to the veterinarian immediately.
3. If the bleeding begins again after you lift the pressure pad, reapply pressure for two additional five-minute intervals. If the bleeding continues, take your pet to the veterinarian. Have someone else drive, if you can, and continue to apply direct pressure en route.
4. When the bleeding has stopped, examine the wound. If it is deep or if the edges are farther apart than one-fourth inch, your pet may need stitches. Take him or her to your veterinarian.
5. If the cut appears to be a minor one, clip the hair around it with scissors and clean the wound with soap and water or hydrogen peroxide.
6. Dry the wound gently.

7. Apply betadyne or wound powder to the injury and bandage it with sterile gauze and tape (see How to Apply a Bandage, Chapter 3). Remove the bandage within twenty-four hours. If the wound is red, painful, or swollen, see your veterinarian. It may be infected and need antibiotics.

Note: Bleeding toenails and small lacerations and scratches can be treated by using a cotton-tip applicator with Pet Stop Bleed, flour, silver nitrate, or other bleed-control compounds.

BLEEDING IN BIRDS

Bleeding in birds is an emergency, since even a small loss of blood can be life-threatening to these animals. First you must restrain the bird and find the source of bleeding. If the bleeding comes from the feathers, pull out the feather and apply clean cotton to the empty follicle using gentle pressure. If a toenail is bleeding, apply a clotting agent such as a silver-nitrate stick, styptic pencil, or flour. Press firmly until the bleeding stops—that is, for five to ten minutes. If the bleeding comes from any other wound, apply gentle pressure directly to the area until the bleeding stops. Then wrap your bird in a warm dry towel and take it to your veterinarian or emergency clinic.

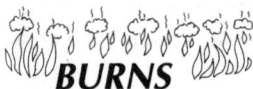

BURNS

Fire, sunlight, friction, or contact with chemicals can cause burns. If your pet has been severely burned and is depressed, he should be seen by a veterinarian as soon as possible.

Symptoms:
1. Redness (indicates first-degree burn)
2. Swelling (indicates second-degree burn)

3. Blistering of skin (indicates second-degree burn)
4. Pain (indicates first- or second-degree burn)
5. Shock.

Treatment:

1. Apply cold water or ice for ten minutes.
2. Dry the area gently with a soft towel.
3. Carefully apply a first-aid cream directly to the wound.
4. See your veterinarian for further evaluation of the burn since shock may occur and antibiotics are sometimes necessary to prevent infection.

Note: *Do not* apply butter or grease to a burn; such treatment can slow the healing process and increase the chance of infection.

CHOKING

Your pet's air can be blocked by any obstruction, such as bones, food, small toys, or pebbles. Immediate first-aid attention on your part is required.

Symptoms:

1. Pawing at the mouth or throat
2. Distress or extreme nervousness
3. Violent coughing or attempts to vomit
4. Loss of consciousness

Treatment:

1. Open the animal's mouth and remove any visible obstruction. Gently pull the tongue out of the mouth to make the throat more visible so you can check for further obstructions. Use a paper

towel or a cloth to grasp the tongue securely. Be careful not to force the object any further down the throat. *Note:* To help protect you from a severe bite, roll the lips over the teeth during this procedure.

2. If you cannot pull out the tongue, pick up your pet by the hind legs and shake him vigorously while slapping his back.

3. As a last resort, try the Heimlich maneuver:
   a. Lay your pet on its stomach. Straddle your pet if it is large.
   b. Put your arms (or hands) around your pet below its rib cage.
   c. Apply a sudden, rapid, upward movement.
   Repeat this process many times until you force out the obstruction.

4. If your pet is still not breathing after the obstruction is removed, clear the airway and administer artificial respiration (see How to Give Artificial Respiration, Chapter 3).

5. See your veterinarian immediately if your pet is having any trouble breathing.

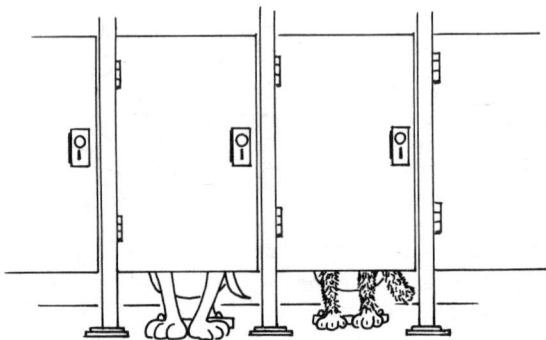

CONSTIPATION

Constipation is more common in older animals and in pets fed an improper diet. Infrequent or difficult elimination of the feces can also result from a loss of intestinal movement caused by disease, spasms, or some abnormality in the nervous system.

Straining to have a bowel movement does not necessarily mean your pet is constipated. It may be a symptom of diarrhea or urinary blockage if only small amounts of urine, mucus, or feces are produced. If you are unsure, see your veterinarian.

Treatment:

1. You can give your pet milk of magnesia, one ounce per twenty pounds of body weight (see Giving Liquid Medication, Chapter 3).
2. If you have no milk of magnesia, you can give your pet mineral oil, two tablespoons per twenty pounds of body weight; the mineral oil can be mixed with the pet's food.
3. Cats can be dosed with one teaspoon of Vaseline placed on the roof of the mouth.

Note: *Do not* give an enema to a cat or dog unless you first check with your veterinarian. An enema may cause poisoning.

DIARRHEA

WARNING: An homogenous, bright-red, bloody diarrhea can be fatal. Take your pet to the veterinarian immediately if this occurs.

Intestinal parasites, viral or bacterial infections, can all cause diarrhea.

Treatment:

1. Give your pet Pepto-Bismol, Kaopectate, or Pet Correct anti-diarrheal medication. Give one tablespoon per ten pounds of body weight every six hours (see Giving Liquid Medication, Chapter 3).

2. Feed a bland diet (cooked rice, strained baby food, boiled chicken) at one-third the normal amount, three times daily (see the recipe outlined below).
3. If your pet is depressed or if the diarrhea lasts over twenty-four hours despite the above treatment, consult your veterinarian. A worm check is helpful, and a teaspoon-sized portion of the diarrhea should be taken to the veterinarian for this purpose.

Note: It is important to have your pet checked for worms several times each year to help prevent problems.

DIET FOR INTESTINAL PROBLEMS

This recipe provides a bland food for the control of diarrhea and/or vomiting caused by diet.

Ingredients:

½ cup Cream of Wheat, cooked (to make about two cups)
1½ cups creamed cottage cheese
1 large egg, hard-cooked
2 tbsp dried brewer's yeast
3 tbsp granulated sugar
1 tbsp corn oil
1 tbsp potassium chloride*
2 tsp dicalcium phosphate*

*Available at local pharmacies and health-food stores.

Directions:

Cook Cream of Wheat according to package directions. Cool mixture. Add remaining ingredients and a balanced vitamin-mineral supplement, such as Unipets or Pet Tabs, and mix well. Yields two pounds, or approximately the amount for a 30-pound dog on a daily basis (two to three meals a day). Can be stored in refrigerator for up to three days. Feed for three to five days—that is, continue to feed for one to two days after the symptoms have disappeared.

Weight of Pet (lb)	Amount of Food (lb)	Amount per Feeding
5	²/₃	Divide total
10	1	portion into
20	1²/₃	2 to 3 equal
40	2²/₃	parts
60	3³/₄	
80	4³/₄	
100	5¹/₂	

DIARRHEA IN BIRDS

Normal bird droppings contain a fecal portion, tubular in shape and dark green or brown in color, and a urinary portion, a combination of white material and water. The water portion can vary, and a watery-looking stool will not necessarily mean that your bird has diarrhea. You will note that the fecal portion is still well formed.

In the case of true diarrhea, the droppings will appear to be like split-pea soup. In that event, administer Kaopectate, adding five to fifteen drops per ounce to the bird's drinking water, depending on the size of the bird. Replace its food with boiled (and cooled) rice water. And take a stool sample and your bird to your veterinarian without delay.

DIARRHEA IN CAGED PETS

Diarrhea in small caged pets can be caused by stress, a change in diet, contaminated water, or infection.

It is indicated by a wetness or dampness around the tail and anus, a loss of form in the droppings, depression or lack of appetite, or a bad odor in the cage.

In the case of diarrhea in a small caged pet, time is your worst enemy. You should act quickly to warm the cage with a 25- or 30-watt lightbulb. Then using an eyedropper, gently feed a mixture of one part Gatorade and one part Kaopectate every two hours until the droppings become firm. (Water can be substituted if there is no Gatorade available.) The proper dosages are given in the table below.

Pet	Amount of Mixture
Mouse	1 cc (¼ tsp.) every 2 hours
Hamster	1 cc (¼ tsp.) every 2 hours
Gerbil	1 cc (¼ tsp.) every 2 hours
Rat	2 cc (⅓ tsp.) every 2 hours
Guinea pig	3 cc (½ tsp.) every 2 hours
Rabbit	3 cc (½ tsp.) per 12 oz body weight every 2 hours

Keep your pet quiet and watch him closely. Additionally feed Veterinarian's High-Energy Formula, honey, or Karo syrup. Consult your veterinarian after twelve hours if your pet is depressed or not eating. If, after twenty-four hours, your pet still has diarrhea, see your veterinarian.

DROWNING

In order to avoid a serious accident, blind, very young, or older pets should be kept away from swimming pools, spas, hot tubs, etc. Should such an accident occur, you must:

1. Pull your pet to safety.
2. If your pet is unconscious, elevate the body so the head will be lower than the rest of the body. Pull the tongue gently out of the mouth until you feel a slight tension and drain any water from the chest.
3. If your pet is not breathing, give artificial respiration by closing the mouth and blowing gently through the nostrils (see How to Give Artificial Respiration, page 50).
4. Take your pet to your veterinarian as soon as possible.

EGG BINDING

If an egg becomes lodged in the bird's cloaca (the chamber at the base of the tail feathers), lubricate the opening with K-Y jelly (or other sterile lubricant) to help your pet expel the egg. Increase the room temperature to 85 to 90°F and, if possible, increase the humidity.

If the bird has not been able to void the egg within twelve hours, consult your veterinarian.

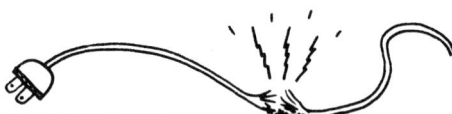

ELECTRIC SHOCK

Some pets, particularly puppies and kittens, are given to chewing on anything at hand. If the object of their chewing should be an electric cord, a serious accident could result.

Symptoms:
1. Difficulty in breathing
2. Burns in and around mouth
3. Loss of consciousness

Treatment:
1. Be careful not to shock yourself. DO NOT TOUCH YOUR PET UNTIL YOU UNPLUG THE ELECTRIC CORD.
2. If your pet is unconscious, give artificial respiration (see How to Give Artificial Respiration, page 50).
3. Because the lungs may fill with fluid, it is important to see your veterinarian immediately.

Note: This condition is not the same as drowning. *Do not* elevate the body above the head and attempt to drain any fluid as this may cause the condition to worsen.

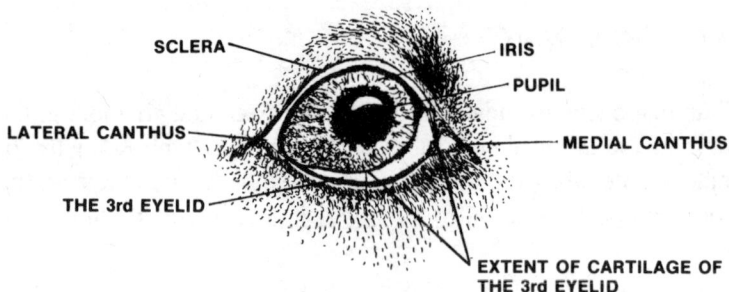

Labels: SCLERA, IRIS, PUPIL, LATERAL CANTHUS, MEDIAL CANTHUS, THE 3rd EYELID, EXTENT OF CARTILAGE OF THE 3rd EYELID

EYE INJURIES AND DISORDERS

Any injury to the eye can be serious, and every eye injury requires an examination. Many injuries to the cornea are not visible without a professional examination. In any event, the primary goal is to help prevent further injury to the eye.

General Symptoms:

1. Squinting and blinking
2. Pawing at the eyes and rubbing the face
3. Discharge, either clear or cloudy
4. Redness and sometimes contraction of the third eyelid

General Treatment:

1. Prevent your pet from pawing or rubbing the eye, but do not struggle to restrain him.
2. If the eyelid is swollen, apply an ice pack to the affected area for five minutes.
3. Pull down the lower eyelid to look for some small foreign object. Flush the eye with a gentle stream of Safe Pet Eyewash, with a contact-lens rinsing solution, or with a commercially prepared saline solution.
4. If you can actually see a foreign object under the upper or lower eyelid but cannot flush it out, use a cotton-tip applicator stick to remove it.

5. If the eye is out of its socket (see Prolapsed Eye below), apply mineral oil or eyewash to the eye every three minutes until you arrive at the veterinarian's office.

SPECIFIC INFECTIONS AND INJURIES

Some specific infections and injuries have unique symptoms and call for professional treatment:

1. *Conjunctivitis* causes a redness of the membranes surrounding the eye. Matter will collect in the corner of the eye, but the eye itself will appear normal. Conjunctivitis is usually treated with an ointment containing cortisone.
2. A *superficial ulcer,* an abrasion or tear in the cornea, will cause your pet to squint or to seem sensitive to light. See your veterinarian.
3. A *deep ulcer* will appear as a concave depression on the surface of the eye. See your veterinarian immediately; keep your pet as quiet as possible until he is examined. *Note:* No ointments containing cortisone should be used in ulcers until healing begins.
4. In the case of a *cut on the eye itself,* see your veterinarian immediately. Keep your pet as quiet as possible and do not use any ointments which contain cortisone in the eye.
5. In the case of a *prolapsed eye* (that is, the eye itself has popped out of its socket), see your veterinarian immediately. There is usually little pain involved with this condition, and the eye can often be replaced in the socket with good results if done as soon as possible. Keep the eye moist with artificial tears or mineral oil if some time must pass before the animal can be examined.
6. In the case of an *enlarged eye,* see your veterinarian immediately. This may be a sign of glaucoma or infection.

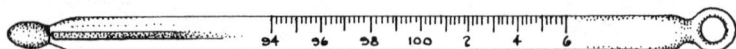

FEVER

Infection, inflammation, heatstroke, pain, or, excitement can cause an increase in your animal's body temperature. (See the table below for normal ranges.)

Normal Body Temperature Ranges*		
Animal	**°F**	**°C**
Cat	100.5–102.5	38.1–39.2
Dog	100.5–102.5	38.1–39.2
Horse	99.5–101.5	37.5–38.6
Mouse	96.4–100.0	35.9–37.8
Hamster†	97.7– 99.5	36.5–37.5
Gerbil	97.5–100.2	36.4–37.9
Rat	99.5–100.8	37.5–38.2
Guinea pig	100.4–102.2	38.0–39.0
Rabbit	102.2–103.2	39.0–39.5
Ferret	100.5–102.0	38.1–39.2

*These are rectal temperatures and must be taken carefully. See How to Take Your Pet's Temperature, Chapter 3.
†In cold weather, hamsters hibernate and can appear to be sleeping or dead, even when perfectly healthy. If your hamster's temperature is below normal, gently warm him in your hands.

Symptoms:

1. Depression and/or inactivity
2. Panting or difficulty in breathing
3. Swelling or painfulness

Treatment:

1. Bring your pet indoors, if practical.
2. Carefully take his temperature (see How to Take Your Pet's Temperature, Chapter 3).

3. If your pet's temperature is above 105°F, see Heatstroke.
4. If your pet is depressed or inactive or if his temperature is elevated, call your veterinarian.

   Note: *Do not* give cats aspirin or any nonaspirin pain reliever.

FROSTBITE

Frostbite occurs most commonly in injured, ill, elderly, or very young pets. It is usually seen on the extremities such as the tips of the ear and the tail.

Symptoms:
1. Pale or reddened skin.
2. Discomfort or pain.
3. Itching.
4. In severe cases, swelling and extreme pain occur, with the affected area remaining cold.

Treatment:
1. Severe cases should be examined immediately by your veterinarian.
2. Warm the affected areas with a warm-water bath for fifteen to twenty minutes.
3. Watch for gangrene (indicated by scabs and darkening of the skin) in the affected areas in the following days.

   Note: See Hypothermia.

HEARTWORM DISEASE

Heartworms are a serious problem in many parts of the United States, especially the South. They are carried from one dog to another through mosquito bites. These worms live in the right chamber of the heart and the large arteries that carry blood into the lungs.

Symptoms:

1. Coughing and gagging
2. Excessive tiring during and after exercise
3. Difficulty in breathing
4. Loss of weight
5. Dull coat and poor condition

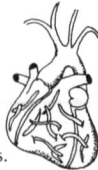

4. Migrate to heart and develop into adult heartworms.

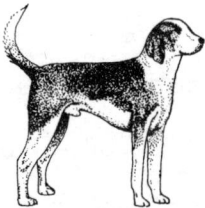

1. Microfilariae (young worms) in bloodstream

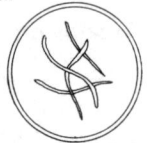

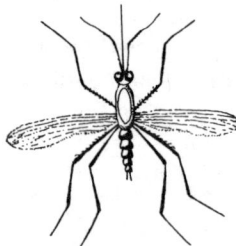

3. Infective larvae deposited under skin when dog bitten by mosquito.

2. Mosquito ingests microfilariae when it bites an infected dog. Microfilariae develop into infected larvae.

Life Cycle of a Heartworm

Treatment:

1. A blood test can be done by your veterinarian to determine if your dog has heartworms.
2. If your dog does not already have heartworms, daily medication can be given to keep him from contracting them. **WARNING:** Do not give heartworm prevention to your pet until he has been checked by your veterinarian. The medication could cause a fatal reaction should he already have heartworms.
3. If your dog has heartworms, your veterinarian will recommend the appropriate treatment considering the animal's age and condition.

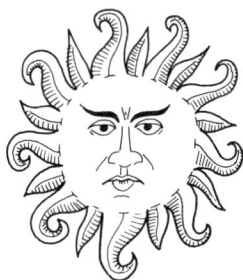

HEATSTROKE

WARNING: Heatstroke can result in death. Heatstroke may happen year-round in warm climates and is typically seen in pets kept in enclosed areas with poor ventilation—in an automobile, a transportation cage, or simply tied up in a yard without proper shade or water.

Symptoms:

1. Rapid, shallow, open-mouthed breathing or panting (Dogs and cats do not perspire as humans do. Their body heat is lost instead through respiration.)
2. A rectal temperature usually greater than 105°F
3. Unconsciousness

Treatment:

1. If you are not sure whether your pet is suffering from heatstroke, carefully take his or her temperature (see How to Take Your Pet's Temperature, Chapter 3).
2. If his temperature is greater than 105°F, immediately immerse your pet's body in cold water until his temperature drops to 103°F.
3. Towel-dry your pet and take him to the veterinarian for further treatment to help prevent permanent brain damage.

HYPOTHERMIA

Many times a pet suffering from frostbite will have an abnormally low body temperature (below 99°F). He could be suffering from a condition called hypothermia.

Symptoms:

1. A low body temperature
2. Excessive shivering
3. A weakened or unconscious condition

Treatment:

1. Wrap your pet in a blanket or other suitable covering.
2. Take your pet indoors out of the cold to warm up.
3. If your pet is wet, use a towel or blow-dryer to dry him.
4. If he is small enough, he may be put against your chest under your shirt.
5. Continue to warm your pet until his temperature is in the normal range. (See table of normal body-temperature ranges given under Fever above.)
6. Hot-water bottles, heating pads, and other safe warming techniques may be used.

7. Weakened animals may be fed syrup or honey and then a warm chicken broth by dropper or syringe.
8. See your veterinarian if your pet continues to be weak or if you suspect frostbite.

   Note: See Frostbite.

INJURIES FROM ENCOUNTERS WITH OTHER ANIMALS

CAT-BITE ABSCESSES

Cats are very territorial and those with access to other cats may fight. Cat bites many times become infected. These infections cause pain and inflammation; the affected area of the body can fill with pus, forming an abscess. *Note:* The wounds are painful and your cat may try to bite while you are examining him.

Symptoms:
1. Depression
2. Loss of appetite
3. Lameness
4. Fever
5. Swelling and pain in an area of the bite, most commonly in the legs, tail, head, or neck
6. A large wound (in the case of an open abscess)

Treatment:
1. Locate the wound; you'll find it in the area that hurts or is swollen.
2. If the wound is draining, clean the area with soap and water or hydrogen peroxide and apply betadyne (povidone-iodine), wound powder, or antibiotic ointment.

3. Often the abscess needs to be lanced, drained, and flushed by your veterinarian. A cat-bite wound is a serious one, and antibiotics will be needed.
4. Keep the wound clean, open, and draining. Do not let a scab form.

Note: These wounds can be a recurrent problem. Having your pet neutered or spayed may help prevent fights.

IMBEDDED PORCUPINE QUILLS

If your pet has been speared by quills, they usually cause pain and can lead to infection.

Treatment:

1. If there are only a small number of quills they can be removed with a pair of pliers. Grasp the quills close to the body and pull out. Do not jerk the quills, break them off, or cut them off in any way. Muzzle your pet if necessary (see How to Muzzle Your Pet, Chapter 3).
2. If there are a large number of quills or if many of them are around the head and face, transport your pet to your veterinarian immediately. (*Do not* let your pet paw at the quills.)
3. Watch your pet for several days. It is possible you have missed some quills; if so, your pet may experience pain, swelling, and infection. Have your pet examined if any of these signs occur.

Note: Many wild animals other than porcupines can be harmful to your pet. Their bites are always dangerous and can be fatal.

SKUNK BITES AND SPRAYS

Skunks are always high-risk rabies suspects; if nothing else their bites can cause infections. And a skunk's spray can severely irritate your pet's sinuses and eyes.

Treatment:

1. You may need the help of another person to carry out the treatment. (If your pet is upset, see How to Approach and Transport an Injured Pet, Chapter 3.)
2. Immediately irrigate the eyes for three minutes with an eyewash, contact-lens solution, or clean water. Put mineral oil in both eyes.
3. Hose your pet with water and wash him with shampoo. Wait five minutes before rinsing. Repeat this procedure twice.
4. While your animal is still wet, pour a solution made of one quart tomato juice and one ounce (two tablespoons) of household ammonia over him. *Do not* rinse off.
5. Allow him to dry in the air, then repeat step 4 two more times.
6. If eye irritation or redness persists or if you suspect your pet may have been bitten, take him to the veterinarian to be examined.
7. Observe your pet closely for the next two weeks for any change in behavior.

Note: Cats will not usually get close enough to a skunk to get sprayed.

ITCHING

Biting insects (fleas, mites, etc.), inhalation of pollens and dust, vitamin deficiencies, and contact with allergenic substances can all cause itching.

Symptoms:

1. Chewing or licking of the feet
2. Rubbing the face or nose with the paws or on the ground
3. Loss of hair
4. Redness, scaling, or scabs on the skin

Treatment:

1. Bathe your pet with a baby shampoo or medicated shampoo.
2. Gently apply a first-aid cream, calamine lotion, or sulfa product to the affected areas.
3. If the itching continues, see your veterinarian for the proper treatment to control the problem and help prevent it from recurring.

LOSS OF APPETITE

Loss of appetite is often a sign that something is wrong with your pet. It does not necessarily mean that your pet is sick. Many times, skipping a meal is a normal thing. There are also seasonal variations in appetite. If your pet skips a meal and is still alert and responsive and shows no other signs of sickness, do not worry. However, if your pet doesn't eat for more than forty-eight hours or shows any signs of sickness—such as pain, depression, or hiding or changes in stool, urination, or breathing—call your veterinarian.

Common causes of appetite loss include:

1. Stress of any kind
2. Fever
3. Upset stomach (Diarrhea, vomiting or gas will usually be present.)
4. Nervousness (Company, a new pet, a new environment, construction noise, thunderstorms, and rain are common causes.)
5. Grief
6. Hot Weather
7. Intestinal blockage (Usually vomiting and gagging occur with this and your pet may look uncomfortable. **WARNING:** This is an emergency. Call your veterinarian if you suspect your pet has eaten something that is not passing.)
8. Internal problems such as kidney failure, liver failure, pancreatitis, inability to urinate, and worms

Treatment:

1. Try to pinpoint a cause from the above list.
2. Call your veterinarian if you have good reason to believe it is anything other than nervousness, grieving, or hot weather.
3. Call your veterinarian immediately if your pet is not alert and active, regardless of the cause.
4. Call your veterinarian if your pet is still not eating after two days, regardless of the cause.

LOSS OF APPETITE IN CAGED PETS

Disease, dirty or contaminated feed and water, improper environment, or stress can cause a loss of appetite in your small pet. You will notice a decreased number of droppings in the cage, and the animal will be seemingly depressed or be in hiding.*

If you note such signs, warm the cage with a 25- or 30-watt lightbulb. Mix one part ground or pelleted feed with one part water and one part Veterinarian's High-Energy Formula, honey, or Karo syrup. Gently try to feed this mixture with an eyedropper at the dosages given below.

Animal	Dosage
Mouse	1 cc (¼ tsp.) every 2 hours
Hamster	1 cc (¼ tsp.) every 2 hours
Gerbil	1 cc (¼ tsp.) every 2 hours
Rat	2 cc (⅓ tsp.) every 2 hours
Guinea pig	3 cc (½ tsp.) every 2 hours
Rabbit	3 cc (½ tsp.) per 12 oz body weight every 2 hours

If, after twelve hours, your pet is worse or no better, see your veterinarian.

---

*Remember that hamsters hibernate. If the cage seems cold, warm your pet slowly in your hands and see if he becomes more active.

PARALYSIS

Paralysis is the partial or complete loss of sensation or voluntary movement in your pet. It can result from an injury, poisoning, infection, or disc disease. If your pet loses its ability to walk or maintain its balance, the condition is generally serious and your veterinarian should be consulted immediately.

Symptoms:

1. Inability to walk or maintain balance
2. Weakness in one or all of the legs
3. Partial or complete loss of sensation (feeling)

Treatment:

Keep your pet as quiet as possible and transport to your veterinarian with care. A rigid board may be used to help carry your pet to your car.

TICK PARALYSIS

Tick paralysis is caused by a chemical produced by certain ticks. The paralysis usually starts in the hind legs and worsens with time until all four legs are involved. **WARNING:** Death can result. If your pet loses its ability to walk or maintain its balance, the condition is generally serious and your veterinarian should be consulted immediately.

Symptoms:

1. Walking weakly and wobbling
2. An inability to rise
3. The presence of one or more ticks on your pet's body (However, the failure to see a tick does not rule out tick paralysis.)

Treatment:

1. Remove all ticks with an approved dip or spray. If there are only a few ticks, you may remove them with your fingers or tweezers. It is best to use a dip after you remove the ticks in case you missed one. Be sure to mark (with lipstick, sticky tape, or Magic Marker) the spots where you removed the ticks for later examination for infection.
2. Take your pet to the veterinarian for further evaluation. Other diseases, such as "coonhound" paralysis may look like this and must be ruled out.

PARASITES, EXTERNAL

FLEAS

Fleas are a problem throughout all regions on at least a seasonal basis; they transmit parasites, including tapeworms, and cause anemia, dermatitis and skin infections, and just plain misery for the pets who are exposed. In severe cases, they can kill your pet.

Control of fleas is a very difficult thing to accomplish; during the "flea season" something will have to be done more than simply a once a week bath if you wish to have effective control. The main thing to remember is that fleas are an environmental problem. Your pet is unfortunately an innocent bystander who is a "grocery store" for these insects. Therefore, an approved spray program for your lawn and house must be initiated, and your pet should be defleaed at the same time. Usually spraying of the environment should be done every two weeks for three to four treatments in order to break the life cycle of the flea. There are many good products available at stores and from veterinarians everywhere. The proper use and precautions, however, must be followed carefully in order to avoid problems with your pets. Birds, fish, and all young animals are more susceptible to pesticide poisoning than are adults.

Symptoms:

1. Scratching, biting, chewing, and licking
2. Loss of hair (especially around the rump and the base of the tail)
3. Whining, crying, or restlessness
4. Red skin with irritation, sores, or scabs
5. Little black specks (flea dirt) in the hair

Treatment:

1. Bathe your pet with an approved flea shampoo.
2. Let the shampoo stay on five to seven minutes.
3. Rinse it off, then let your pet sit in cool, fresh water for five minutes.
4. Call your veterinarian for more information on the best flea control method for your area.

Note: If you don't have flea shampoo you can temporarily use dish soap or your own shampoo as a substitute. Also, Avon's Skin So Soft and Lemon Fresh Joy can be used until the appropriate flea medication can be purchased.

TICKS

Ticks are a seasonal problem and are commonly found in fields and woody areas. They can cause skin problems and anemia from blood loss and are known to transmit many diseases to humans and animals. (See Tick Paralysis above.) There are many dips, powders, and sprays to kill them. If you are in an infested area, weekly baths and dips for your pet will be required, with careful watch in between. *Note:* Check with your veterinarian before using any new chemical on your pet, and always read the label on any insecticide carefully before use.

Symptoms:

1. Presence of ticks anywhere on body, but most commonly around the neck and ears

2. Weakness or staggering
3. Itching, localized sores, or irritation

Treatment:

1. Spray your pet with approved spray.
2. Bathe or dip your pet.
3. Call your veterinarian.

Note: Be careful removing ticks, since it is easy to leave a part of the tick while pulling the insect off your pet. Mark the area with a Magic Marker or a lipstick so that you can immediately identify the area for your veterinarian.

PARASITES IN BIRDS

Birds are particularly vulnerable to external parasites. Should you notice any abnormal growth on the beak, cere, or legs or an increase in the loss of feathers or in the bird's picking at its feathers, take it to your veterinarian for proper diagnosis and medication.

PARASITES, INTERNAL

COCCIDIA AND GIARDIA

Coccidia and giardia are microscopic protozoan parasites that may cause diarrhea. They are treated like worms.

WORMS

Worms can be very serious if allowed to go untreated. The most life-threatening are not visible to the eye, so periodic microscopic fecal checks by your veterinarian are important. *Note:* Puppies and kittens are especially susceptible to worms and intestinal parasites and should always be checked.

Symptoms:

1. Diarrhea and/or vomiting
2. Blood in the stool
3. Weight loss
4. Dull coat and poor condition
5. Anemia

Treatment:

1. Take a portion of your pet's feces to your veterinarian to determine what kind of worms your pet has.
2. Treat with the proper medicine. For some of the more serious worms, there is no effective treatment sold over the counter. It is important to check with your veterinarian if you worm (deworm) your pet yourself.

The most common worms are discussed below (see also Heartworm Disease above).

HOOKWORMS

Though they are invisible to the human eye, these parasites can be very serious, often causing diarrhea and sometimes causing death in puppies and occasionally in adult pets. Hookworms are very common in the South; they can be contracted from the mother animal or from walking on contaminated ground and then licking the feet.

ROUNDWORMS

Roundworms are especially common in young animals; they are off-white in color, are generally two to five inches long, and are seen in the pet's vomitus or stool. Young animals contract round-worms from their mothers, or from walking on contaminated ground and then licking their feet.

Over-the-counter wormers are often effective for roundworms, but check with your veterinarian first to be sure your pet does not have any other type of worms.

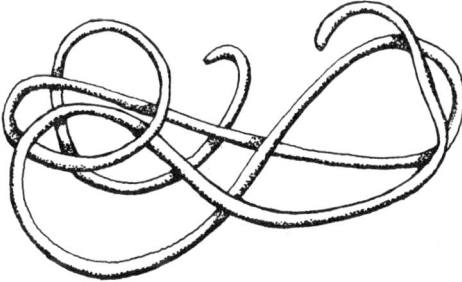

TAPEWORMS

Tapeworms, carried by fleas and rodents, are generally not as serious as other worms. They are off-white in color, are one-fourth to four inches long, and are flat. They are usually seen around the base of your pet's tail. When dry, they appear like grains of rice and are usually seen in the pet's bedding.

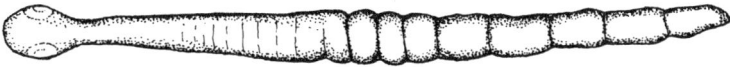

WHIPWORMS

These parasites can cause chronic diarrhea, vomiting, or lack of appetite. Though invisible to the naked eye, they can be serious and are contracted by walking on contaminated ground and then licking the feet.

PARASITES IN BIRDS

Birds are particularly vulnerable to internal parasites. Symptoms of infestation include vomiting, diarrhea with or without blood, and constipation or a decrease in the number of droppings. If you observe any of these signs, take a stool sample and your bird to your veterinarian for diagnosis and medication.

Note: Routine stool checks are recommended for young birds; for birds over one year of age, a stool specimen should be examined every six months.

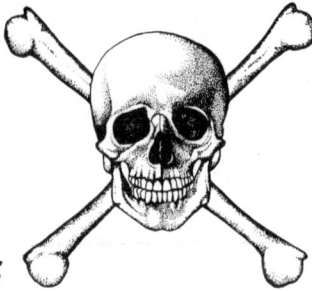

POISONING

Pets are very curious and care should be taken to keep them away from harmful products and medicines. (See tables below.) If you think your pet has been poisoned, call your veterinarian immediately. **Note:** If you are told to bring your pet in, take the container of any product suspected of poisoning him. This will help your veterinarian know what the antidote might be.

Treatment for Poisons Taken Internally (by mouth):

1. If the poison has caused sores or swelling to your pet's mouth or tongue, do not induce vomiting. Do not induce vomiting if your pet is unconscious or if he has swallowed strychnine; corrosives such as alkalies (lye) or strong acids; or petroleum distillates such as kerosene, gasoline, coal oil, fuel oil, paint thinner, or cleaning fluid. Call your veterinarian or the poison-control center if there is any question.

2. When vomiting is indicated (see Common Pet Poisons), it can be induced by giving any of the substances listed below. Hydrogen peroxide is the method of choice. Save any vomited material. It may help your veterinarian identify the poison.
3. If your pet is excited or having seizures, move him to a soft surface and transport him to your veterinarian immediately.

SUBSTANCES TO INDUCE VOMITING

Animal	Hydrogen Peroxide	Salt	Dry Mustard	Syrup of Ipecac*
Cat	1 tbsp.	½ tsp.	½ tsp.	2 tsp.
Small dog, 15 lb or less	1 tbsp.	½ tsp.	1 tsp.	2 tsp.
Medium dog, 16–40 lb	2–3 tbsp.	1 tsp.	2 tsp.	1 tbsp.
Large dog, 41–80 lb	4 tbsp.	2 tsp.	1 tbsp.	2 tbsp.

*Takes thirty minutes to work.

Treatment for Poisons on Skin or Fur

If your pet has been poisoned by something on its skin or fur, wash him with soap and water repeatedly and check with your veterinarian for further treatment. Apply first-aid cream to any burns or irritations.

COMMON PET POISONS

Poison	Induce Vomiting?	Poison	Induce Vomiting?
Acetone	Yes	Furniture polish	No
Alkalies	No	House plants	Yes
Alcohol, all types	Yes	Insecticides	Yes
Antifreeze	Yes	Lead	Yes
Ant poisons	Yes	Lye	No
Arsenic	Yes	Malathion	Yes
Aspirin (cats)	Yes	Matches	Yes
Bleach	No	Mushrooms	Yes
Burnt lime	No	Pencils	Yes
Carbon monoxide*	—	Pine oil	No
Chemicals	No	Rat poison	Yes
Cleaners	No	Shoe cleaner	Yes
Crayons	Yes	Shoe polish	Yes
Diazonon	Yes	Spoiled food	Yes
Dichlorvos	Yes	Tar	No
Drugs	Yes	Tylenol (cats)	Yes
Fertilizers	No	Warfarin	Yes

*Give artificial respiration. (See How to Give Artificial Respiration, Chapter 3.)

POISONING IN BIRDS

Birds love to chew, especially things that are new to their environment. But many things are poisonous to your pet, including plants, lead, and foreign objects. *Note:* Overheated teflon pans create vapors that are deadly to birds.

Signs of poisoning in a bird include vomiting, diarrhea, lethargy, difficulty in breathing, and depression.

If you observe such symptoms, see your veterinarian as soon as possible for crop flushing.

POISONOUS PLANTS*

Amaryllis	Dumbcane	Philodendron
Autumn crocus	Foxglove	Poinsettia
Bagpod	Horse chestnut	Poppy
Bitterweed	Hyacinth	Rattlebox
Bleeding heart	Iris	Rhododendron
Box hedge	Ivy, English	Rhubarb
Buckeye	Jasmine	Sleepy grass
Castor bean	Jimsonweed	Snowdrop
Cherry laurel	Lantana	Solanum (night shade)
Chinaberry	Larkspur	Sneezeweed
Christmas rose	Laurel	Tobacco (in flower)
Cocklebur	Lily of the valley	Tung oil tree
Copperweed	Lupine	Water hemlock
Crotolaria	Milkweed	Wheat
Death camas	Mistletoe	Yew
Diffenbachia	Oak bud	
Dry maria	Oleander	

*Induce vomiting for all these plants.

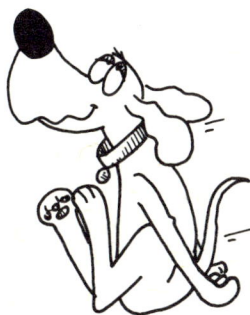

SCOOTING

Scooting is often caused by impacted or infected anal sacs, allergies, fleas, or worms.

Symptoms:
1. Dragging the hind quarters along the carpet or grass
2. Licking or chewing around the anus

Treatment:
1. Gently lift your pet's tail and look for any irritation around the anus.
2. If the area is irritated, carefully apply a first-aid cream.
3. If there is no apparent irritation or if there is no improvement after treatment, take your pet to be examined.

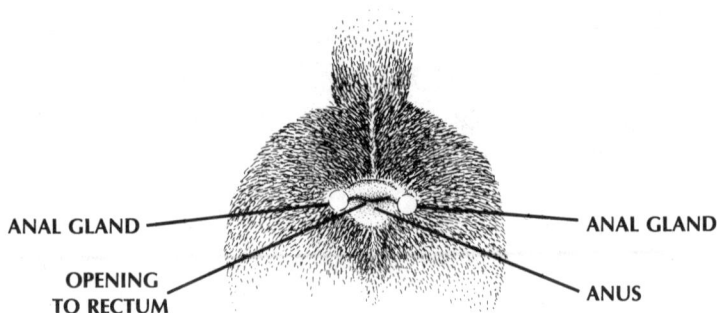

ANAL GLAND —————————————— ANAL GLAND

OPENING TO RECTUM —————————— ANUS

SEIZURES

Poisons, a blow to the head, a birth defect, or internal disease can cause seizures. All seizures should be reported to your veterinarian so that the proper diagnosis and treatment can be determined.

Symptoms:
1. In a grand mal seizure, your pet will be lying on its side with the legs kicking and the head and neck extended. This condition usually lasts one to two minutes, and your pet may experience a period of confusion following the seizure.
2. A mild seizure can be evidenced by an inability to recognize people or by any unusual behavior.

Treatment:

1. Leave your pet alone to recover on its own unless it is in a place where it can be hurt. If your pet must be moved, do not put your hands near its mouth because it is possible for an animal having a seizure to bite without knowing it is doing so.
2. Take your pet to the veterinarian immediately if the grand mal seizure lasts longer than four minutes or if your pet has several seizures in a row.
3. Take your pet's temperature (see How to Take Your Pet's Temperature, Chapter 3). If the temperature is greater than 105°F, see Heatstroke and follow treatment.
4. If your pet is unconscious and not breathing, administer artificial respiration (see How to Give Artificial Respiration, Chapter 3).

Note: If your pet is pregnant or a nursing mother, the seizure may be due to a low level of calcium in her blood. Take her immediately to your veterinarian for treatment.

If the seizure occurs during or after exercise or after a period of not eating, your pet could be suffering from hypoglycemia (low blood sugar). Give honey, Karo syrup, or Veterinarian's High-Energy Formula at the following dosage:

Small pet	½ tsp
Cat or small dog	1 tsp
Medium dog	1 tbsp
Large pet	2 tbsp

Seizures in Birds

Seizure in a bird is indicated by uncontrolled behavior; that is, the animal is observed thrashing around its cage and flapping its wings in an agitated manner. These seizures can last from fifteen seconds to three to five minutes.

Wrap your bird in a towel and use gentle restraint until the seizure ends. Care should be taken to avoid being bitten, especially by a large bird such as a parrot. Once the bird is alert and calm again, give small amounts of sugar, Karo syrup, or honey water. Consult your veterinarian.

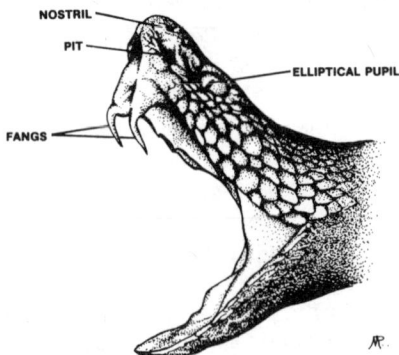

SNAKEBITES

Any poisonous snake, alive or dead, can be dangerous. Exercise extreme caution.

Signs and Symptoms
1. Two fang marks (slashes or punctures)
2. Immediate pain in the area of the bite. Be careful when you feel the wound. Your pet may bite as a reflex to this pain.
3. Rapid swelling
4. Bleeding and oozing from the wound
5. Dark blueish-purple discoloration in the skin around the bite wound
6. In severe cases, depression, vomiting, loss of balance, and convulsions may occur.

Treatment:
1. Rush your pet to the veterinarian or nearest veterinary emergency clinic. Antivenom is available and must be given as quickly as possible.
2. Identify the snake, but don't endanger yourself.

If you are unable to reach your veterinarian or veterinary clinic within one hour:

1. Keep your pet calm.
2. If at all possible, carry him instead of letting him walk.
3. If he or she has been bitten in the leg, apply a snug Ace bandage or gauze wrap directly above the wound area, being careful not to cut off all circulation.
4. Apply an ice pack directly to the bite area and OVER the Ace bandage.
5. Take your pet to the veterinarian immediately. Drive carefully.

SNEEZING OR COUGHING

Periodic sneezing or coughing is not an emergency in most animals. If it is prolonged or seems bothersome to the pet it should be checked, since it may be indicative of choking, poisoning, worms, or some other pathologic condition.

SNEEZING IN BIRDS

Birds sneeze two or three times daily as a part of their normal behavior. More frequent sneezing could be indicative of trouble. Provide the bird with fresh food and water and increase the cage (or environmental) temperature to 85 to 90°F (see discussion under Trauma below). If there is no improvement in twelve hours, consult your veterinarian.

TRAUMA

In case of any accident your pet may experience trauma. (Trauma in the primary sense is the injury itself. Here we speak of it as both the injury itself and the shock resulting from the injury.) Calm the animal, treat any apparent physical injury and observe his behavior. Shock can be fatal. Consult your veterinarian immediately. (See also Accidents earlier in this chapter.)

TRAUMA IN BIRDS

Trauma in birds is an especially critical condition.

1. First check for hemorrhaging; if bleeding is discovered, use the first-aid techniques described under Bleeding earlier in this chapter.
2. Check the bird's wings. If one is broken, tape both wings loosely to the body and keep the bird quiet. If a leg is broken, do not attempt treatment; simply keep the bird quiet. *Note:* More damage can be done trying to apply a splint to a bird than by leaving it alone.
3. In the event of any injury, keep the bird quiet. Cover the cage or place him in a cardboard box. Keep him warm (85 to 95°F), using one of three methods:
    a. Place the cage on a heating pad with the control set low and cover the cage with a light blanket.
    b. Use a 25- to 30-watt lightbulb placed in a box and put in the cage. Be sure the bulb is not close enough to burn the box or the bird.
    c. Put a space heater in the bathroom and warm the room to 85 to 90°F. A thermometer placed near the cage will help you monitor the cage temperature. **WARNING:** *Do not* allow the cage temperature to exceed the recommended level.

URINATION DIFFICULTIES

Infection in the bladder or kidney, bladder or kidney stones, inflammation of the urethra, irritation of the vagina or penis, and prostate problems in the male can cause straining to urinate. The most serious consequences occur when your pet is unable to urinate at all, usually because of stones blocking the urinary tract. **WARN-ING:** Straining to urinate should always be considered an emergency.

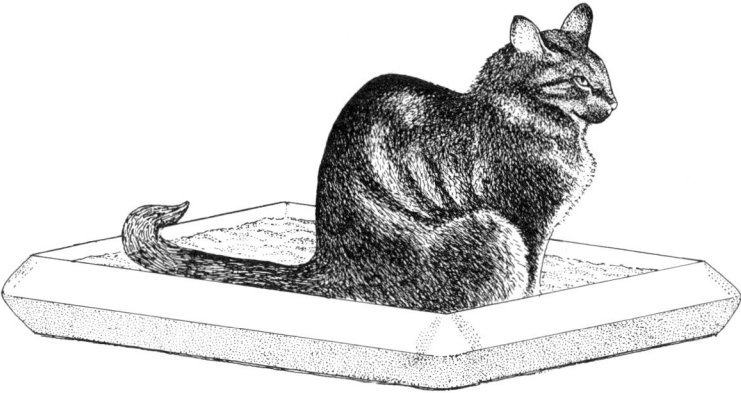

Symptoms:

1. Repeated attempts to urinate in an unusually short period of time.
2. An expression or sound of pain when your pet urinates.
3. Any abnormal appearance of the urine (bloody, dark, cloudy, etc.).
4. Small amounts of urine, or no urine at all, expelled.
5. Moving to several areas in an attempt to urinate.
6. In the most advanced state, your pet may not be able to stand and will have a swollen abdomen; vomiting may occur.

Treatment:

1. Take your pet to the veterinarian immediately for an examination since the situation could be life-threatening, especially in males.
2. Antibiotics, urinary acidifiers, salt, or a special diet may be prescribed for your pet.

VOMITING

Eating spoiled food or a substance irritating to the stomach often causes vomiting. Table scraps and garbage are two common culprits.

Treatment:

1. Withhold all food and water for several hours. If the vomiting continues or if your pet becomes depressed or inactive, see your veterinarian as soon as possible.
2. If there is no vomiting for two hours, give your pet a small amount of crushed ice to lick.
3. If there has been no vomiting for four hours, give your pet one-fourth to one-half cup of water every hour.
4. If there is no vomiting for twenty-four hours, feed a bland diet—cooked rice, strained baby food, or boiled chicken (remove the skin and bones)—at one-third his normal diet amount every six hours. (See the recipe given under Diarrhea earlier in this chapter.)
5. If the vomiting becomes a recurrent problem, contact your veterinarian.

WARNING: Sometimes vomiting can be a sign of bloat. Bloat is a condition characterized by a distended abdomen, vomiting, pain in the abdomen, or dry heaving. This is an emergency. Your pet can go into shock and die. Time is very important. Large-breed, deep-chested dogs are most susceptible, though bloat can occur in any pet. Never feed large meals and then exercise your pet.

VOMITING IN BIRDS

Birds often regurgitate to mates or to other birds as a sign of affection. They may also regurgitate in front of a mirror or when being greeted by their owners. This is normal. Abnormal vomiting, on the other hand, is indicated by forced, uncontrolled regurgitation wherein the bird spews the food around its cage. In abnormal vomiting, too, regurgitated food will collect on the head feathers.

Should you notice any signs of abnormal vomiting you must take your bird to the veterinarian.

CHAPTER THREE

PRACTICING FIRST AID

HOW TO ASSEMBLE A PET FIRST-AID KIT

To be prepared for most any emergency involving your pet you should have a first-aid kit. Commercial kits are available from your veterinarian or pet-supply store or you can put one together yourself. Below is a list of items we recommend for a first-aid kit. Ask your veterinarian to recommend other products specifically for your pet's needs.

1. Plastic box or fishing-tackle box
2. Adhesive tape, 1 in wide
3. Gauze bandage roll, 3 in wide (2 in wide for small pets)
4. Sterile gauze pads, 3 × 3 in
5. Scissors
6. Splint (e.g., tongue depressor or 12-in wooden ruler)
7. Pet Correct, Kaopectate, or Pepto-Bismol
8. 3% hydrogen peroxide
9. Antibacterial ointment (povidone-iodine, bacitracin, or triple antibiotic ointment)
10. Antibiotic powder, povidone-iodine, or furacin
11. Vitamin A & D ointment
12. Silver-nitrate sticks, styptic pencil, or Pet Stop Bleed
13. Boric acid eyewash, Safe Pet Eyewash or other eyewash containing 0.9 to 2% boric acid
14. K-Y jelly or other sterile lubricant
15. Chemical ice pack or plastic freezer bags for ice
16. Tweezers
17. Pet Lax or mineral oil

18. Thermometer
19. 12-cc syringe for oral medication
20. Eyedropper
21. Karo syrup or Veterinarian's High-Energy Formula
22. Q-tips or sterile cotton-tip applicator sticks
23. Wire cutters or needle-nose pliers
24. Betadyne or wound powder

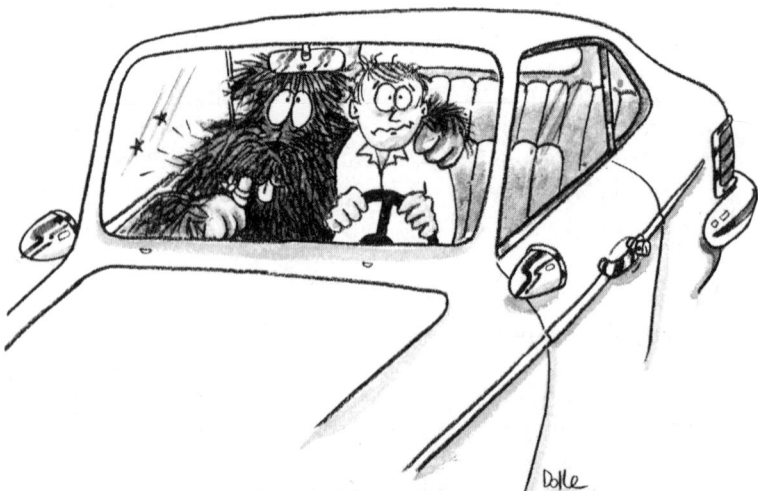

HOW TO APPROACH AND TRANSPORT AN INJURED PET

APPROACHING AND TRANSPORTING CATS

While talking in a soft, calm voice, approach the cat very slowly. Leisurely lower your body and gently pet the cat behind the head and between the ears. Begin to pet the rest of the head and neck if the cat is still calm. Slowly pick the cat up by reaching over the shoulders and under the chest. Bring him or her slowly under your arm. Hold the front legs with one hand and the head and neck with the other while snuggling the cat against your body with your elbow.

Note: If the cat is hissing or spitting, do not attempt to pick him up without protection. Drop a blanket (or a towel or pillow cover) over the cat, then scoop the blanket under the animal and pick him up.

If the cat cannot move, place him on a board or piece of stiff cardboard and secure him to the "stretcher" with strips of cloth or soft rope.

APPROACHING AND TRANSPORTING DOGS

Dogs should be approached in a manner similar to that described above. Talk softly and watch for any signs of aggression such as growling, snarling, or a wide-eyed appearance. If you have the animal's confidence, place a rope, leash, or three layers of gauze around his neck. If the animal is in pain or if you are unfamiliar with him, muzzle the dog (see How to Muzzle Your Pet below). If you must pick him up, place one hand in front of the shoulders below the neck and the other under the rump, behind both back legs. Pick him up slowly.

If the dog can't walk, use a board or other flat, sturdy object. If it is a small dog, a piece of stiff cardboard may be used. Secure the dog to the stretcher and transport him to the veterinarian.

Note: Do not attempt to transport injured wild animals. Unless you have had experience, call your county animal-control unit, Humane Society, or other animal-welfare organization.

HOW TO MUZZLE YOUR PET

You should muzzle your dog whenever you attempt to handle him in a way that may cause or increase pain. Even the best-tempered dog may bite in reflex to the pain.

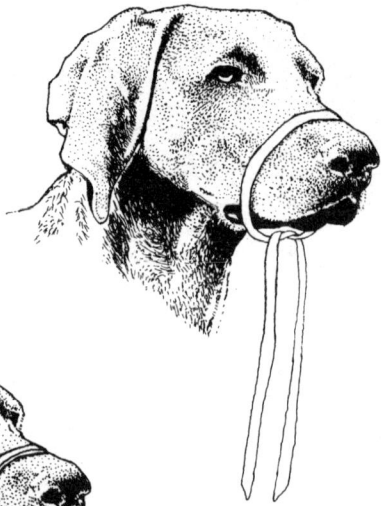

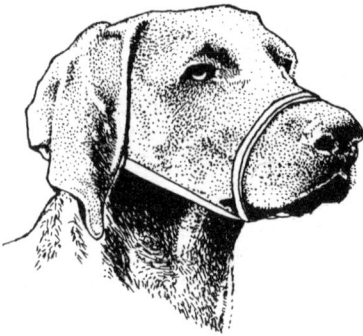

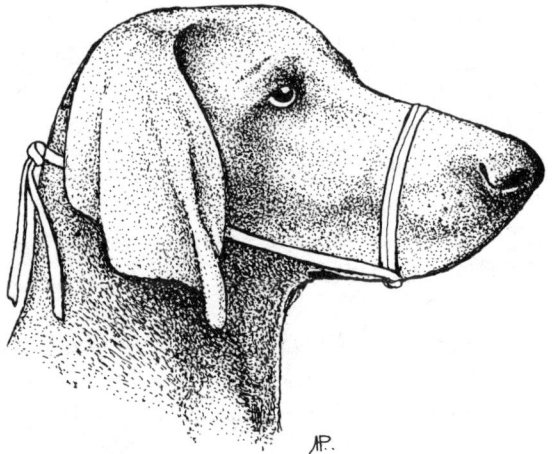

1. Wrap a gauze bandage or soft rope around the snout, placing it about half way up the nose. Tie at least two times.
2. Loop the bandage or rope from under the chin to behind the ears; tie a double knot.

Note: The muzzle should be tight enough so that your pet cannot open his mouth; however, it must be loose enough to enable him to breathe through his nose. He should not be struggling for oxygen (see facing page). Remove the muzzle immediately should this occur.

HOW TO GIVE ARTIFICIAL RESPIRATION

When giving artificial respiration to an animal, be sure his mouth is clear of all foreign material. Cup your hands around the muzzle to prevent air from escaping. (You may have to place your mouth completely over the nose of your pet.) Blow gently into the nostrils, at a rate of eight to ten breaths per minute. You should see the chest rise. Let if fall back naturally. Continue this procedure until a breathing response or coughing occurs.

Note: See also How to Give Cardiopulmonary Resuscitation below (see illustration on page 52).

HOW TO GIVE CARDIOPULMONARY RESUSCITATION (CPR)

Cardiopulmonary resuscitation is sometimes necessary in case of severe injury. This procedure is difficult even for experienced technicians. Do the best you can.

1. Place the animal on his right side on the ground or on a table.
2. Check for a heartbeat by pressing your fingers firmly against the lower side of the animal's chest immediately behind the elbow.
3. If there is no heartbeat and your pet is not breathing, begin CPR:

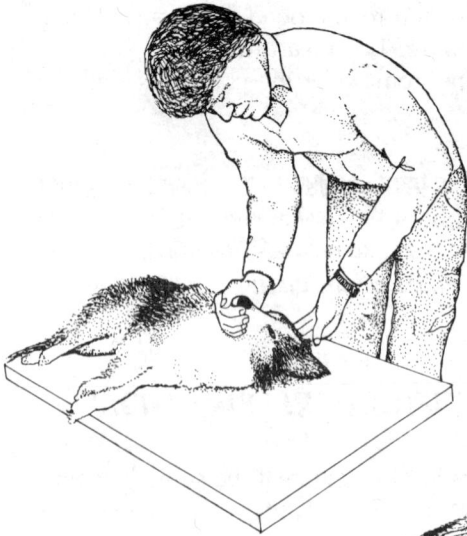

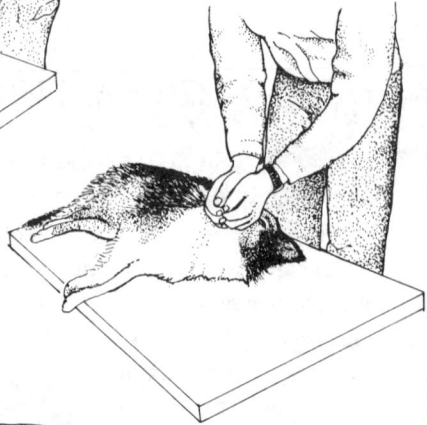

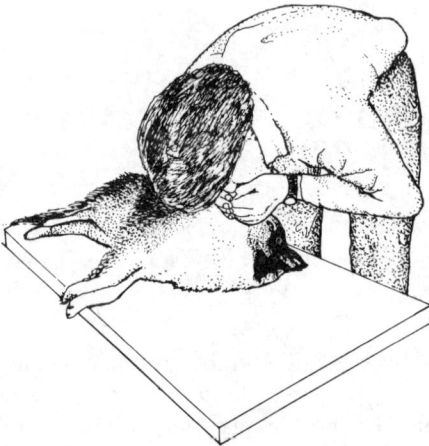

a. Pull the tongue out to make sure you have an open airway.
b. With your pet lying flat, place the heel of your hand on the chest behind the elbow in the brisket area (see Anatomy of the Dog, Chapter 7). If your pet is large (forty-five pounds or more), it may take both hands.
c. Rapidly compress the chest six times, allowing one to two seconds between compressions.
d. Give three breaths by artificial respiration. (See How to Give Artificial Respiration above.)
e. Repeat chest compression six times and feel for the heartbeat. If there is still no beat, repeat three breaths of artificial respiration.
f. Continue the procedure for five minutes or until the heart begins and your pet is breathing.
g. If after five minutes there is still no heartbeat, have someone drive you and your pet to the nearest veterinarian. Continue the CPR procedure while en route.

HOW TO STOP BLEEDING

Bleeding from a cut or wound can generally be stopped by applying direct pressure. First obtain a clean cloth or sterile gauze pads to cover the wound.

1. Place the cloth or gauze directly over the bleeding area.
2. Apply direct pressure just firmly enough so that the bleeding stops. Continue to apply pressure for five minutes.
3. Remove the pad and make sure the wound has stopped bleeding. If the bleeding continues, repeat the procedure. (See treatment outlined in Bleeding, Chapter 2.)

For bleeding toenails take a cotton applicator stick and place Pet Stop Bleed or flour on it. Press firmly against the nail for three minutes. Silver-nitrate sticks or a styptic pencil can also be used. If

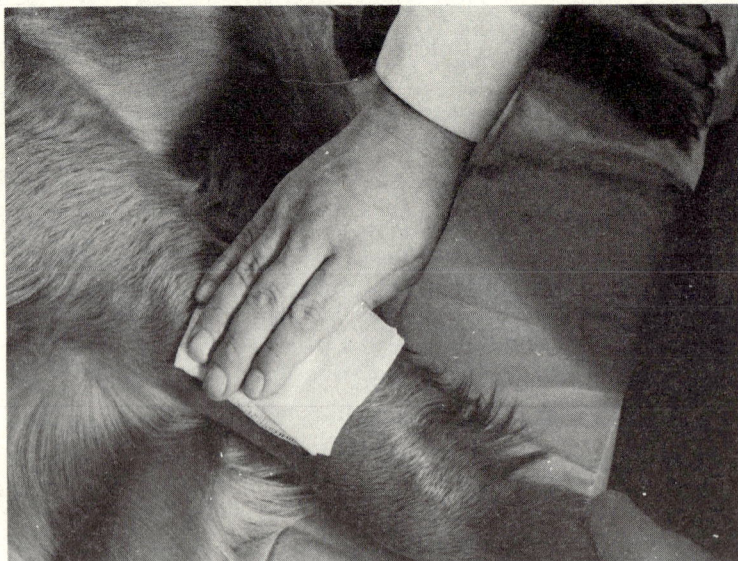

(1)

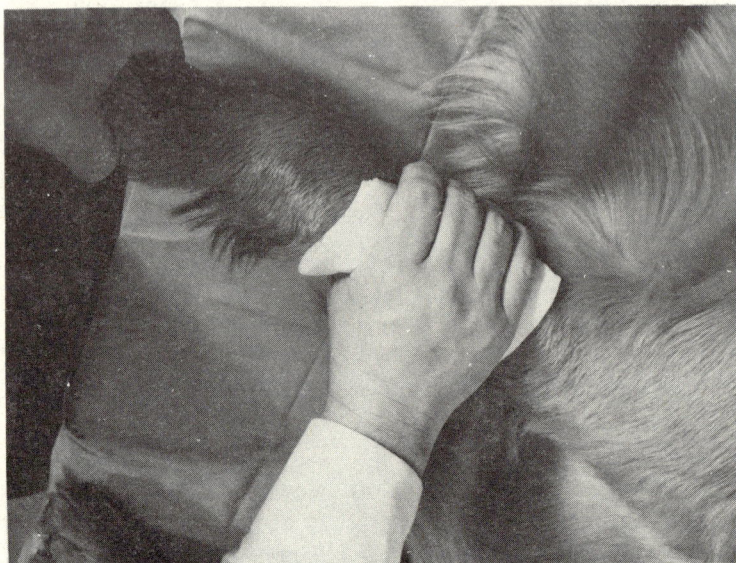

(2)

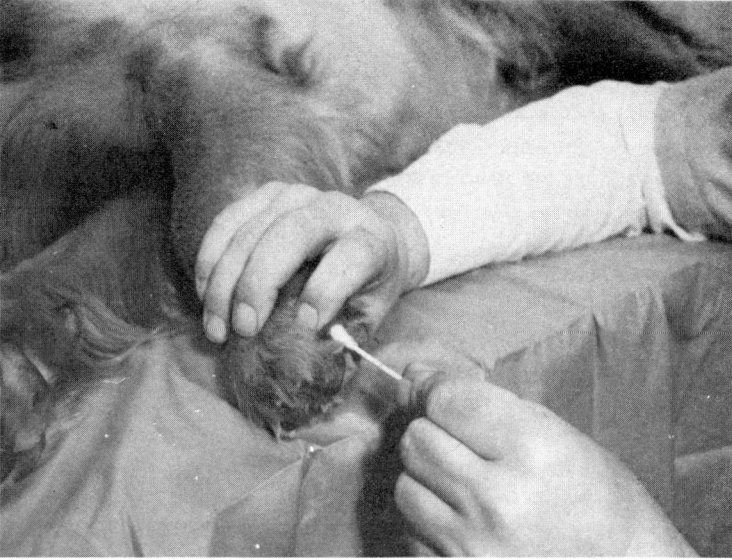

(3)

bleeding continues, lightly roll applicator back and forth while still applying pressure.

Note: If the bleeding cannot be controlled within fifteen minutes continue to apply direct pressure and transport the animal to your veterinarian.

HOW TO APPLY A BANDAGE

BANDAGING A LEG

The pain from an injury could cause your pet to bite. Before bandaging the injured leg, it may be necessary for you to muzzle him. (See How to Muzzle Your Pet earlier in this chapter.)

1. Identify the wound. If it is not clean, wash it gently with soap and water. Apply betadyne, wound powder, or an antiseptic to the wound.

2. Place a clean gauze pad—sterile, if possible—over the wound.
3. Roll on several layers of gauze or cast padding so it is snug, but not tight. It is better to have the bandage too loose than to cut off your pet's circulation.
4. Leave the toes uncovered.
5. Now apply tape; start to roll it on above the elbow and above the padding or gauze so the bandage will be anchored securely.
6. Continue to roll the tape down the leg. Again, be very careful not to make the bandage so tight as to interfere with the leg's normal circulation.
7. Leave the toes uncovered.
8. While the bandage is on your pet, check it at least every twelve hours for slippage or soiling. It is *very important* to check the toes for swelling. If swelling should occur, remove the bandage immediately.
9. Remove the bandage in twenty-four hours and rebandage only if necessary. If pain, swelling, or drainage is present, take your pet in for an examination.

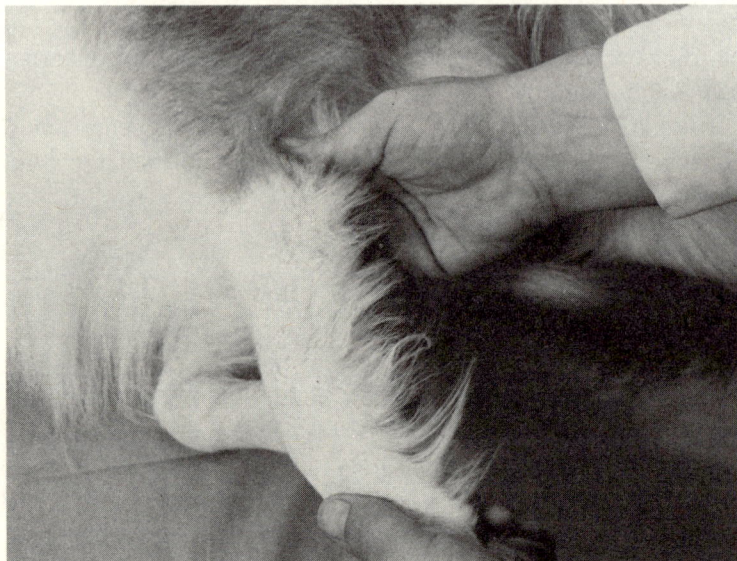

(1)

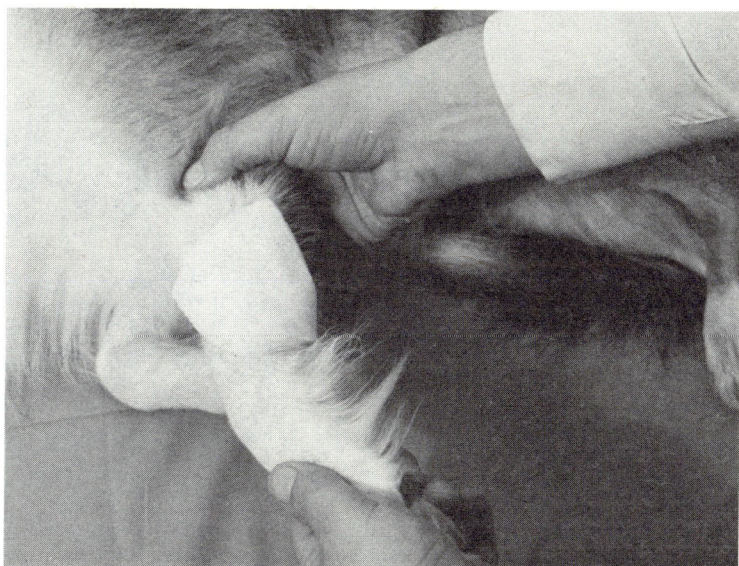

(2)

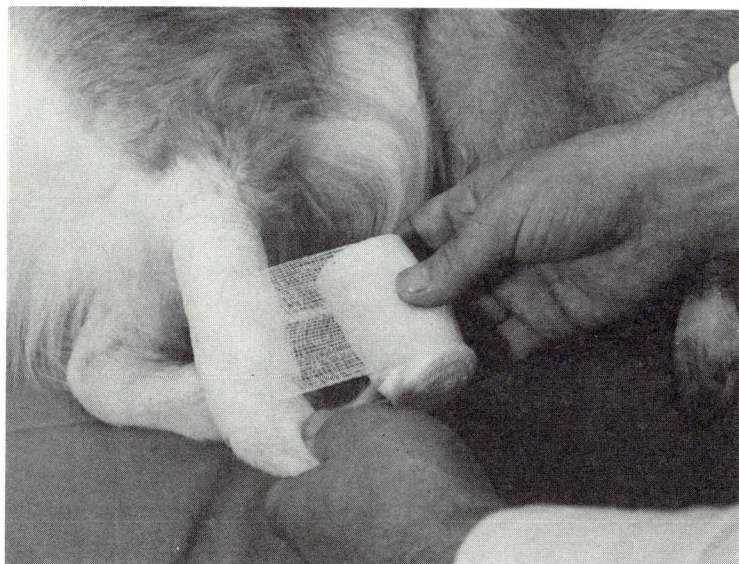

(3)

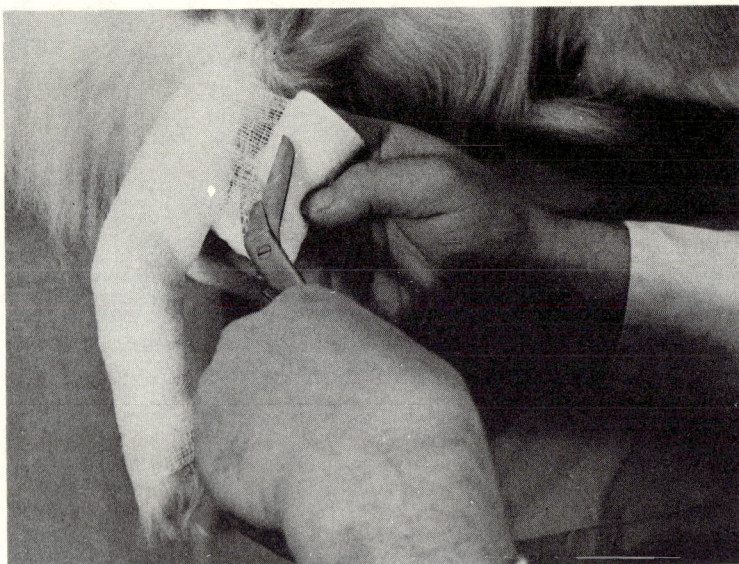

(4)

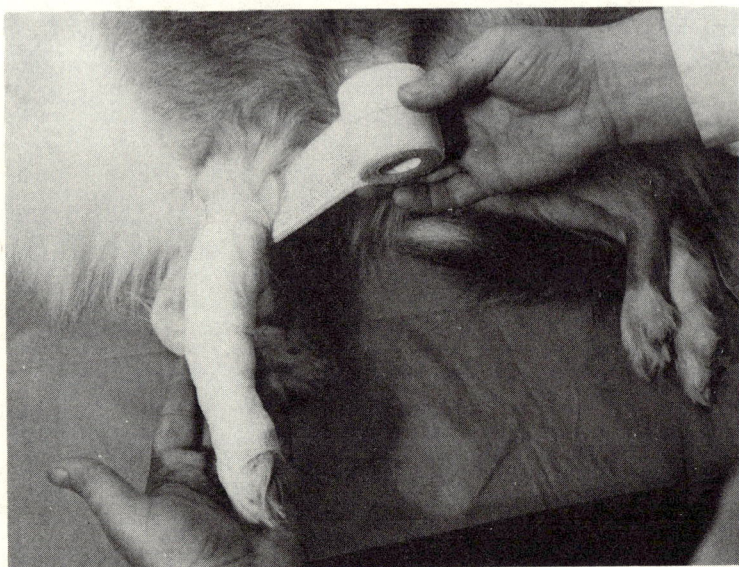

(5)

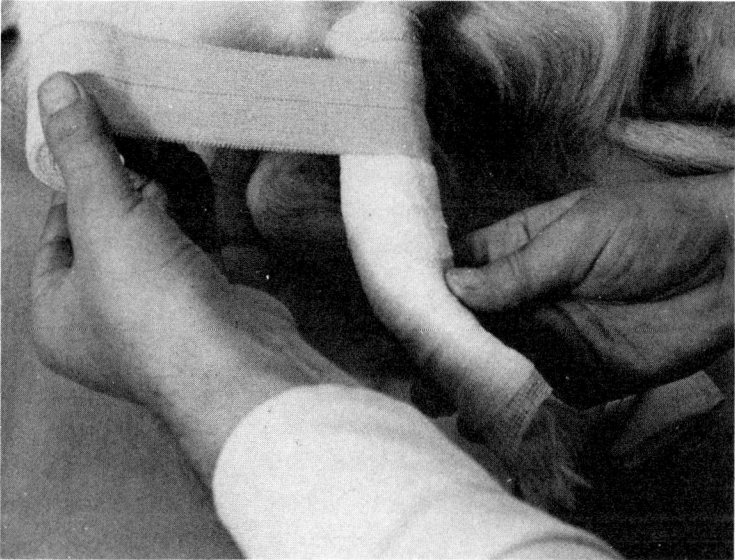

(6)

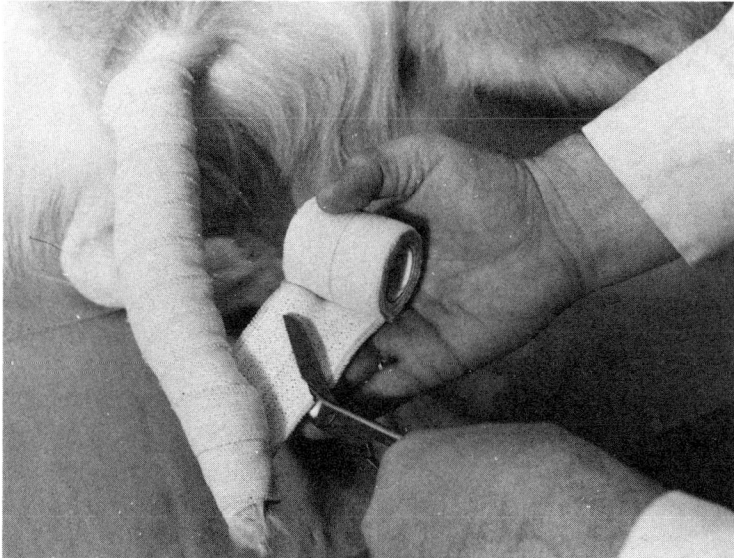

(7)

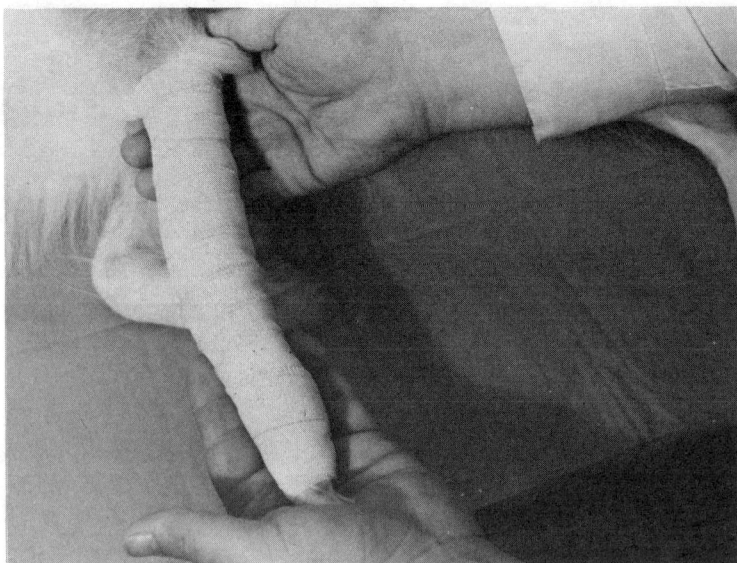

(*8*)

BANDAGING THE CHEST OR BODY

It is especially important to wrap the chest when you hear sucking noises through a wound. See your veterinarian as soon as possible because this means the chest cavity has been penetrated. If there is a severe injury to the abdomen, the technique illustrated below can be used to apply a body bandage. Remember, it may be necessary to muzzle your pet before proceeding to bandage him. (See How to Muzzle Your Pet earlier in this chapter.)

1. Place a clean pad—sterile, if available—over the wound.
2. Begin taping across the gauze pad so it will be anchored securely to your pet's body.
3. Wrap the tape around the chest, taking care the bandage is not so tight as to interfere with normal breathing movement.
4. The tape should extend several inches on either side of the gauze pad.

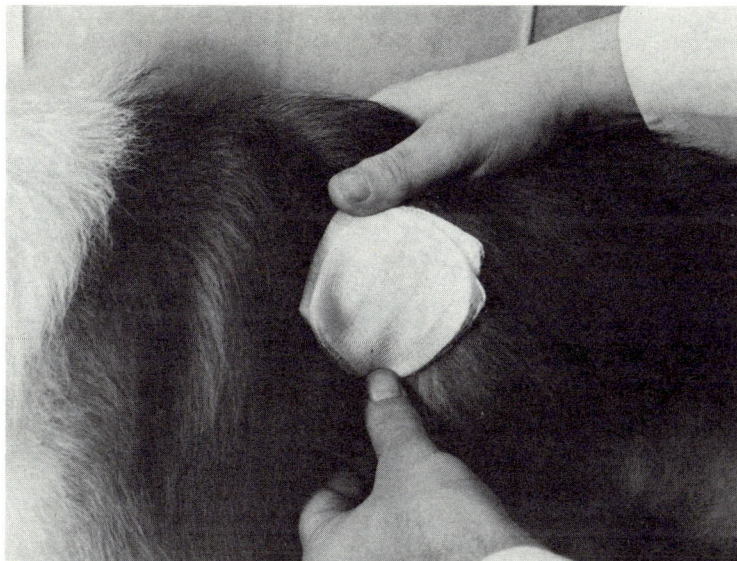

(1)

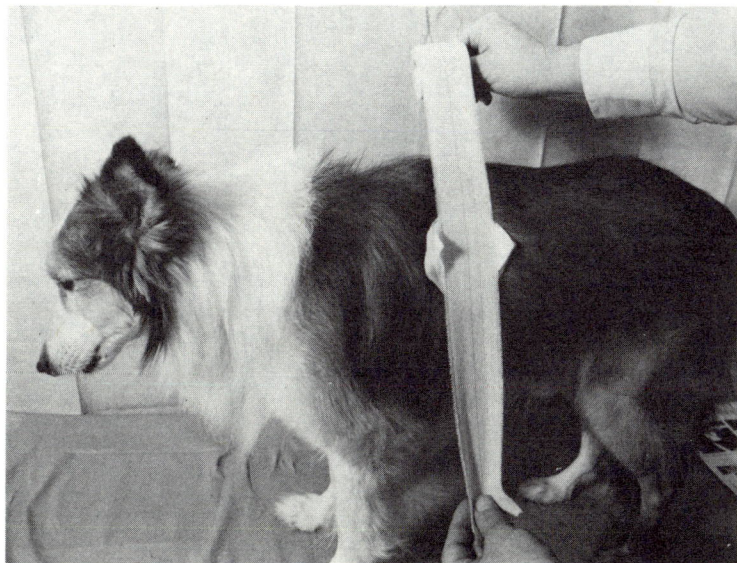

(2)

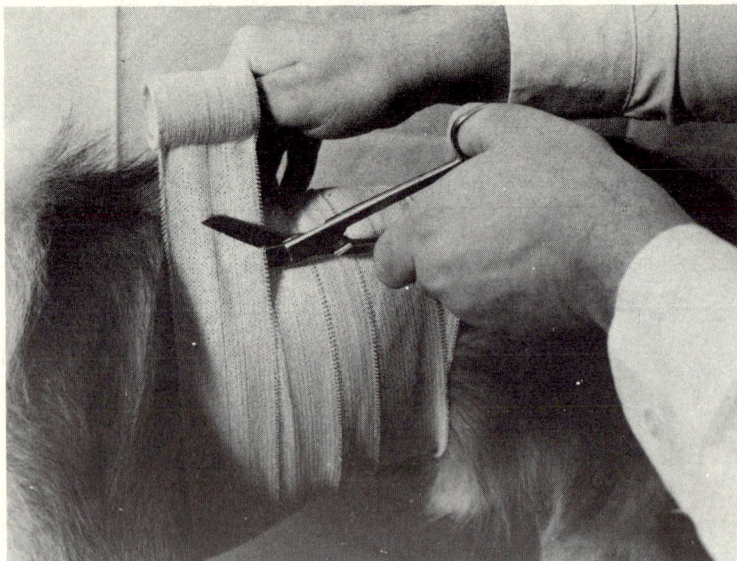

(3)

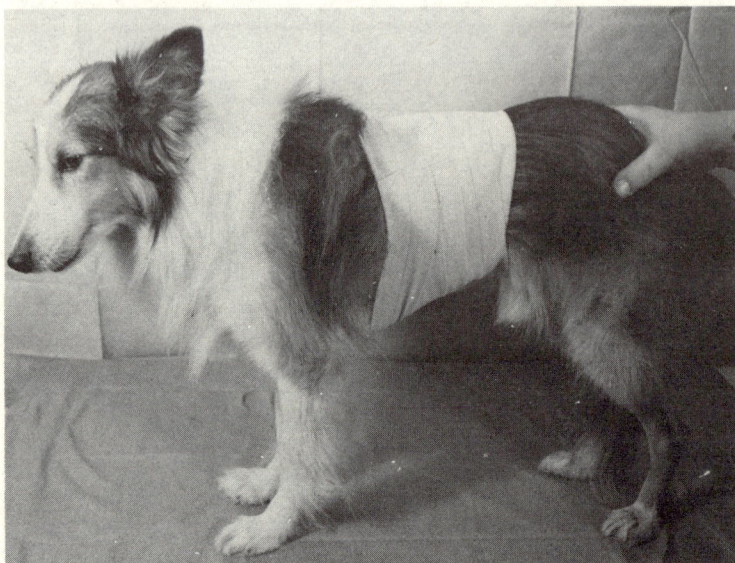

(4)

HOW TO APPLY A SPLINT

Pain can cause your pet to bite as a natural reflex, so it is advisable to muzzle him before applying a splint (see How to Muzzle Your Pet earlier in this chapter).

1. Keep the limb straight by bracing it at the elbow; do not pull on the foot. Place a thick magazine under the leg.
2. Loosely roll the magazine around the animal's leg, then place a piece of tape around it.
3. Begin taping at the top, above the elbow, so the splint is securely attached to the leg.
4. Continue taping down the leg.
5. Do not cover the toes.

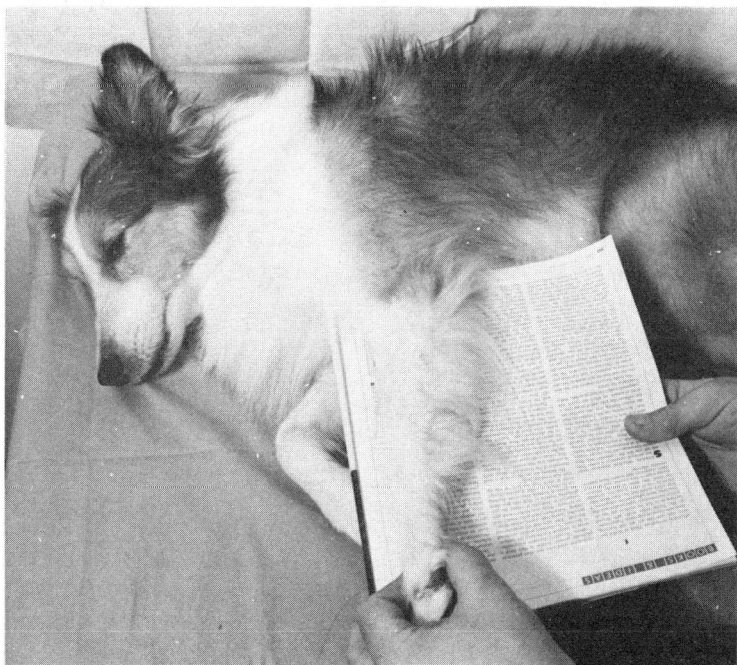

(1)

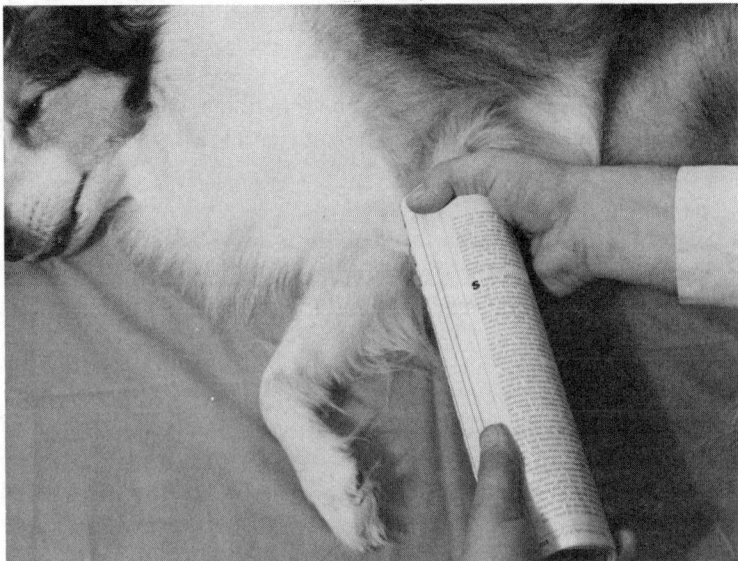

(2)

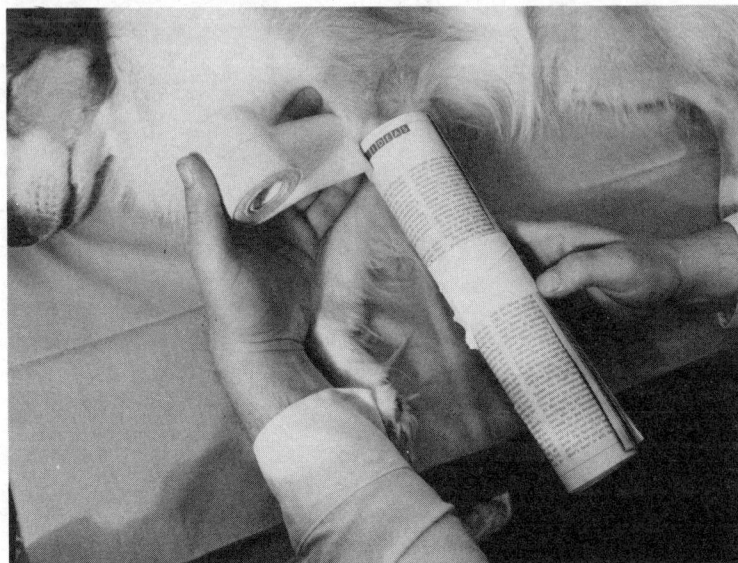

(3)

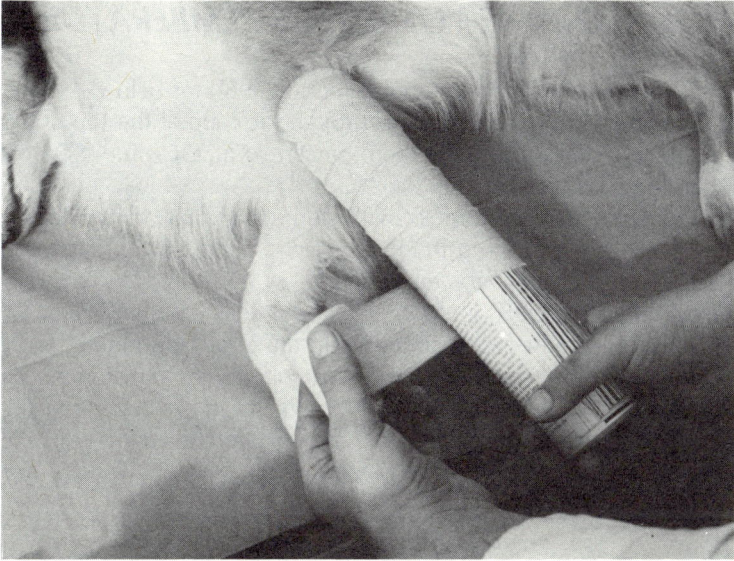

(4)

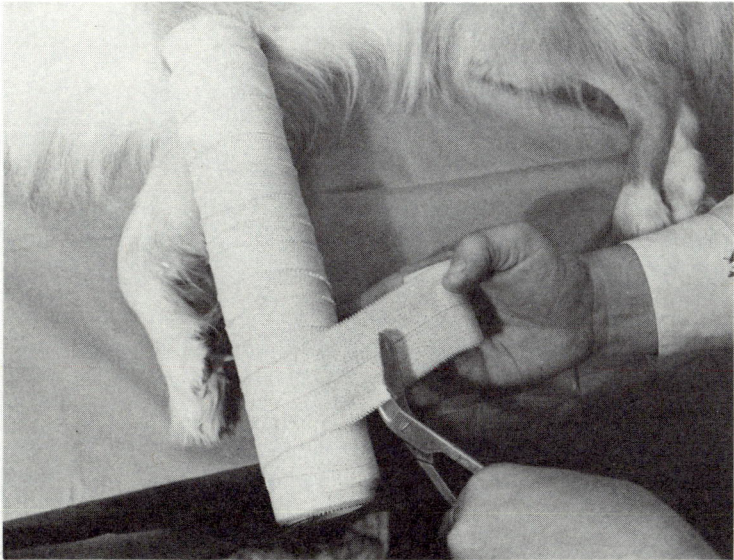

(5)

HOW TO TAKE YOUR PET'S TEMPERATURE

1. Shake the thermometer until it registers 96°F or below.
2. For safety, either tie a string through the loop at the top of the thermometer or hold the thermometer so that it will not be lost in the rectum.
3. Lubricate the thermometer with sterile lubricant or Vaseline.
4. Lift the tail and insert the thermometer gently into the rectum. *Do not force so as to cause pain.*
5. The thermometer should be inserted at least one-half its length into the rectum and should remain there for two minutes.
6. Remove the thermometer and wipe off any fecal material with a wet paper towel. Hold the thermometer in the horizontal position and look between the numbers. Rotate slowly until the mercury column becomes visible.

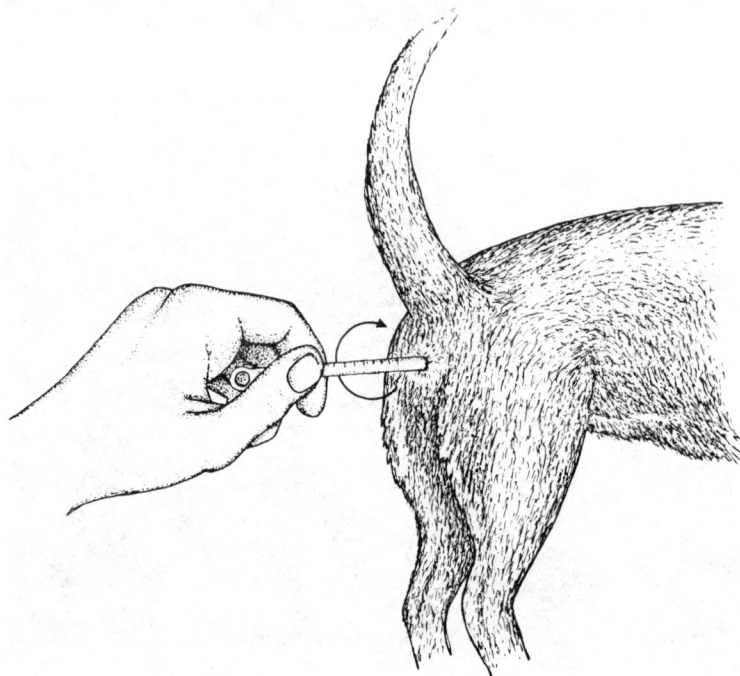

The normal temperature range of your pet can be found under Fever, Chapter 2. Once you know your pet's normal temperature, you will be able to evaluate how much fever the animal has. At times you may think your pet is running a fever because he feels hot, his nose is dry, or he is quiet and not acting right. But those conditions do not necessarily indicate fever.

Note: It is often difficult to take the rectal temperature of small caged pets, kittens, or puppies. Have your veterinarian show you how to do this if you are not experienced, since you could hurt your pet.

HOW TO GIVE MEDICATION

GIVING LIQUID MEDICATION

Use an eyedropper or syringe to administer liquid medication.

1. Hold your pet's head at a 45° angle. Pull the back corner of the lip down and place the dropper or syringe in the corner of the mouth (see illustration on next page).
2. As he swallows, slowly administer the liquid.
3. Keep the mouth closed until all the liquid is down.
4. You may rub the throat to help stimulate swallowing.

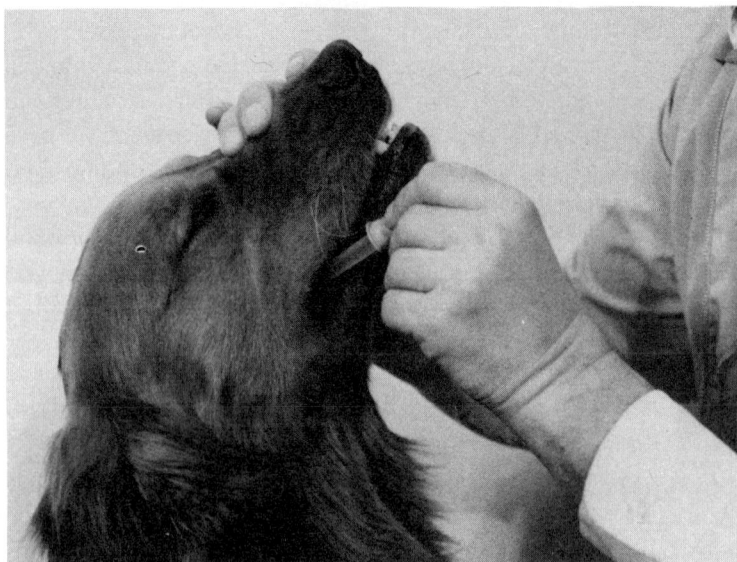

(1)

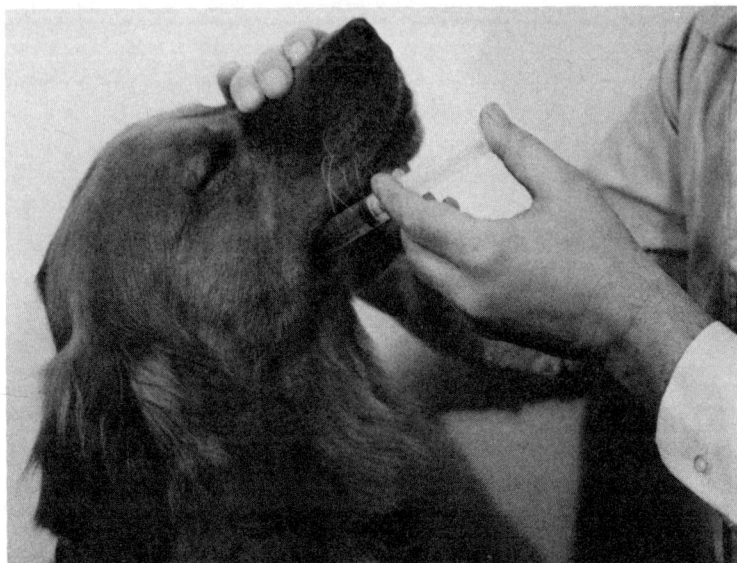

(2)

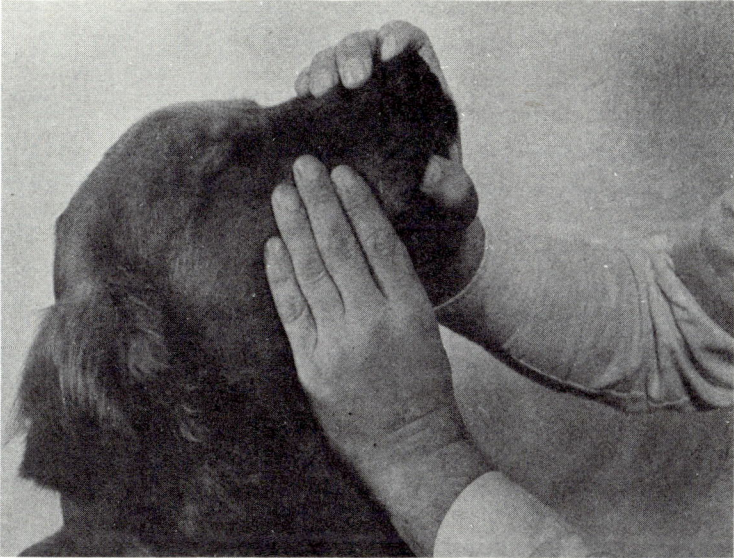

(3)

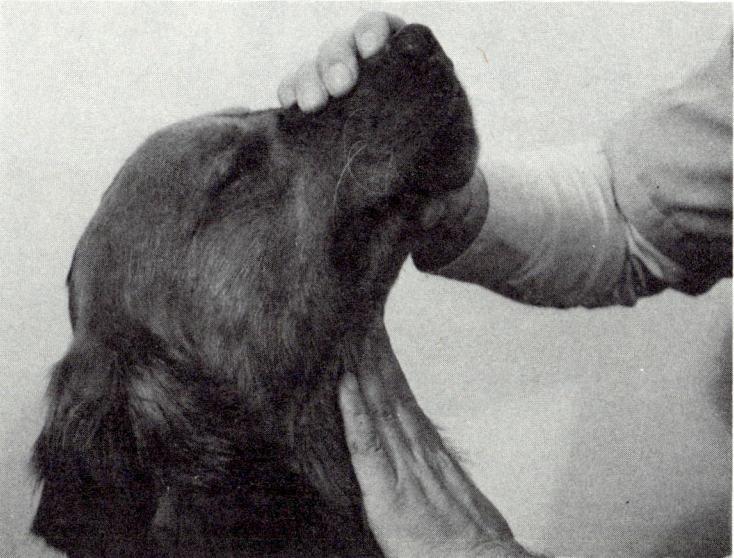

(4)

GIVING CAPSULES, PILLS, OR TABLETS

1. Your pet should be in a standing or sitting position with his head at a 45° angle.
2. Hold the pill between the thumb and forefinger of your left hand (or whichever hand is more comfortable).
3. While pushing the upper lips over the teeth with your right hand, use the last three fingers on the left hand to open the lower jaw.
4. Insert the pill into the mouth as much in the center and as far back as possible.
5. Quickly close the mouth and rub the throat and nose gently to stimulate swallowing.

Note: The pill can be coated with butter to make it taste better and easier to swallow.

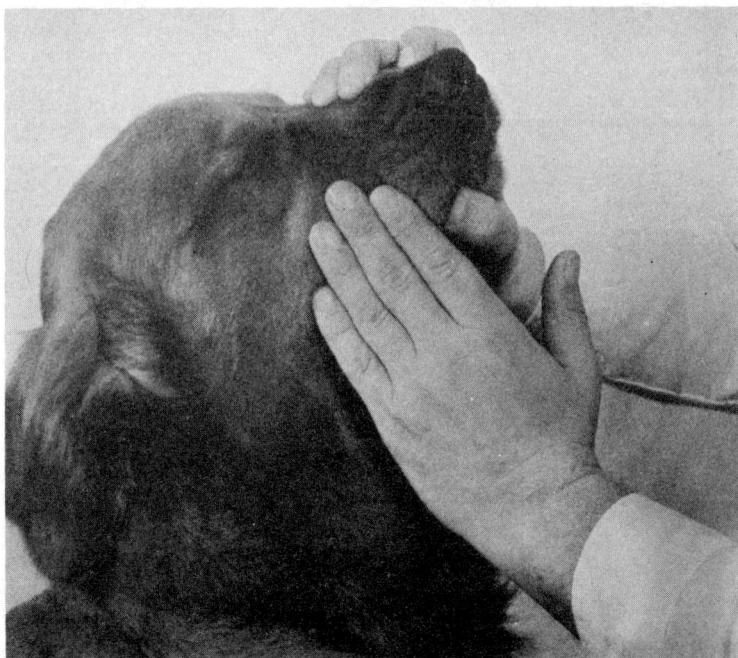

(1)

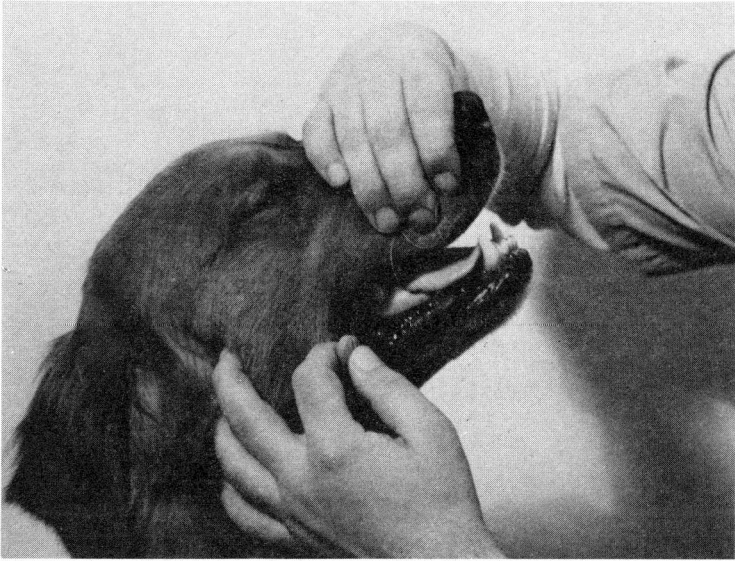

(2)

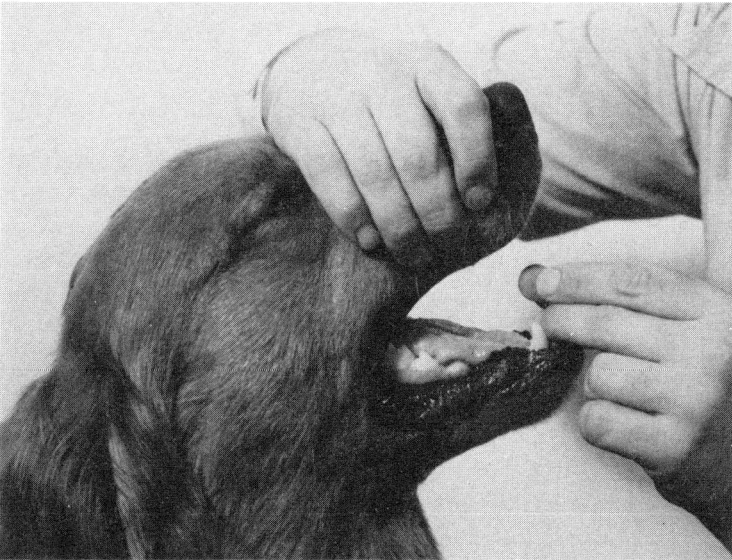

(3)

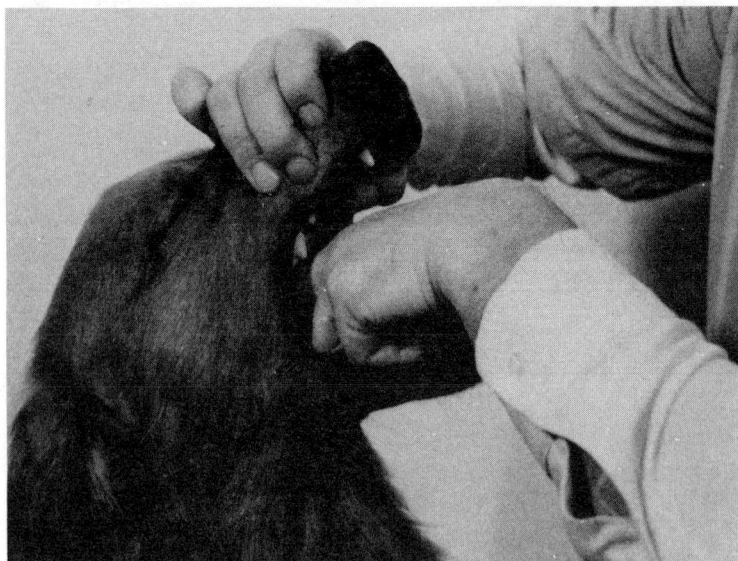

(4)

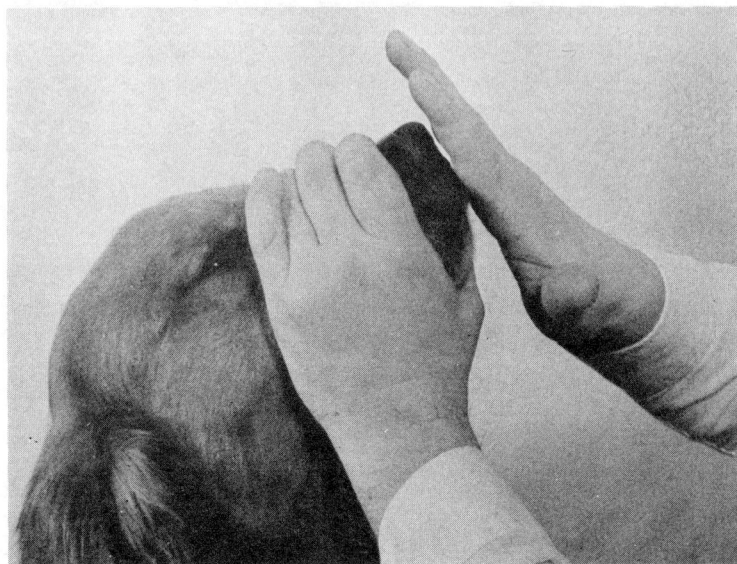

(5)

AN ALTERNATIVE METHOD

1. Your pet should be in a standing or sitting position with his head at a 45° angle.
2. Move your thumb behind the canine tooth (fang) and onto the roof of the mouth.
3. Press upward against the roof of the mouth.
4. Insert the pill into your pet's mouth as far back and as much in the center as possible.
5. Close the mouth quickly.
6. Rub the throat and nose gently to stimulate swallowing.

It is often difficult to give a pill to a cat. Check with your veterinarian for assistance. If your cat is easygoing and you can open his mouth without getting bitten or scratched, coat the pill with butter, drop the pill into the mouth as far back and as close to the center of the tongue as possible. Close the mouth quickly and hold it closed; rub his nose. When your cat licks, the pill has been swallowed.

Note: Do not struggle with your pet as this will make matters worse.

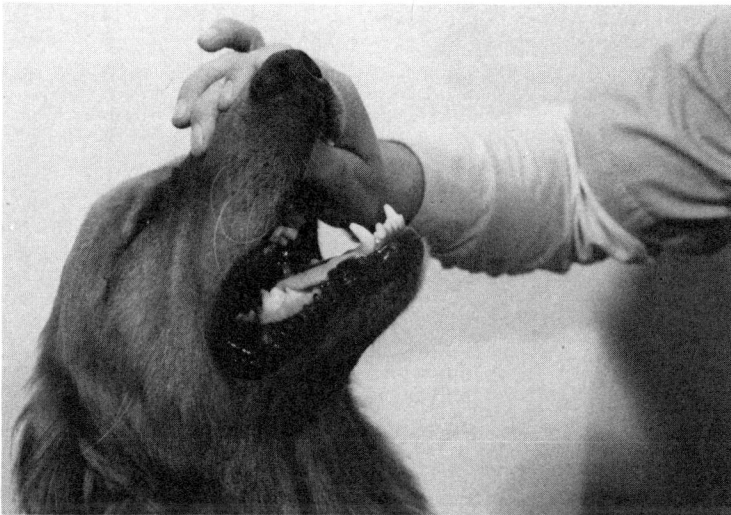

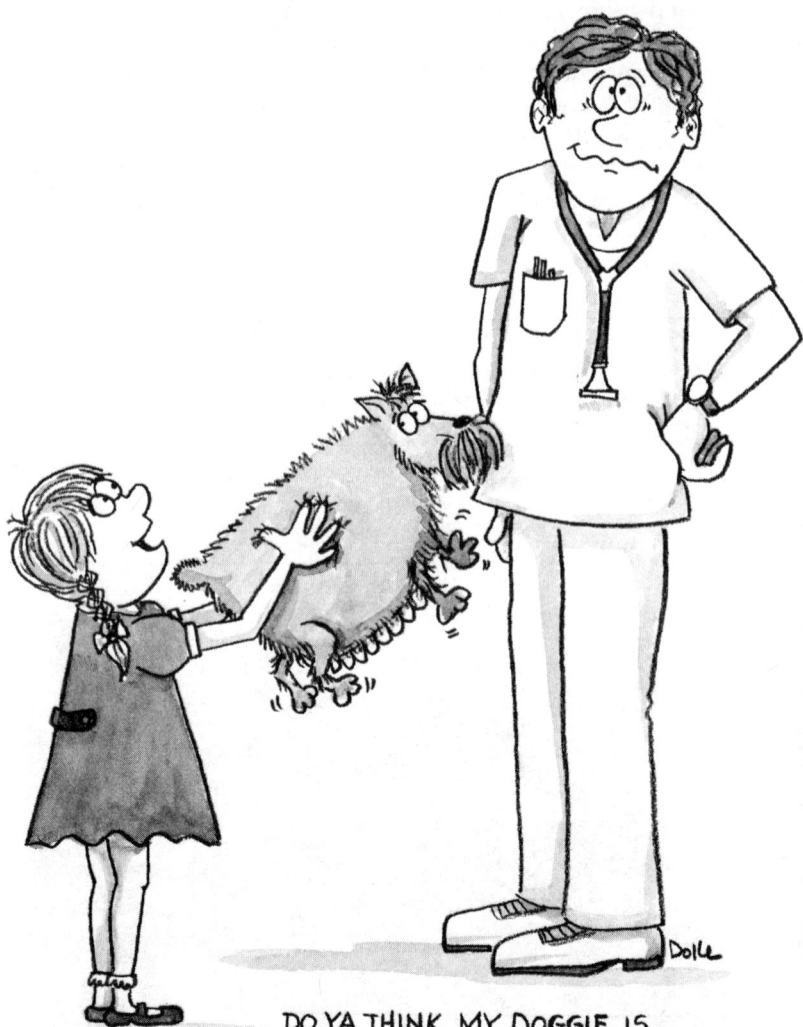

DO YA THINK MY DOGGIE IS
PREGNANT, DOCTOR?

CHAPTER FOUR

NEUTERING, BREEDING, AND BIRTHING

SPAYING OR NEUTERING YOUR PET

If you do not intend to breed your pet, you should have the animal spayed or neutered, not only to prevent "surprise" litters but also to help protect his or her health and attractiveness as a pet.

The reasons for having the procedure done are many. Unspayed or unneutered pets can be aggressive toward other animals of the same sex. This is especially true of tomcats. Unneutered males may roam to find a female in heat, thus exposing themselves to accidents of many kinds. Both sexes, unaltered, are also prone to mark their territory (your house or your yard) by periodic urination, a malodorous habit.

The medical reasons for spaying or neutering your pet are very sound. These procedures eliminate risk of certain types of cancer. Neutering greatly decreases the chance of prostate trouble in male animals, and spaying prevents serious, life-threatening infections in the uterus of females. In addition, it eliminates the risk of a type of diabetes found in older female dogs.

Spaying or neutering is usually done when the animal is between six months and one year of age; check with your own veterinarian for his or her recommendation.

If your animal is accidentally bred, talk to your veterinarian about the advisability of giving her a shot to abort the pregnancy. For the greatest success, the injection should be given as close to the breeding as possible—that is, within one to three days.

BREEDING INFORMATION

Animal	Time in Heat	Interval between Periods of Heat	Gestation Period, days	Breeding Age	Age at Puberty
Gerbil	12–18 h	4 days	24–25	12 wk	9–12 wk
Guinea pig	5–18 h	16–19 days	65–72	14 wk	8–10 wk
Mouse	9–20 h	4–5 days	19–21	8 wk	5–7 wk
Rat	9–20 h	4–5 days	21–23	14 wk	6–9 wk
Hamster	4–24 h	4–5 days	16–18	8 wk	4–7 wk
Rabbit	2 wk	14–16 days	32	7 mo	5–7 mo
Dog	15–21 days	Half year (spring and fall)	58–63	1½ yr	6–9 mo
Cat	4–10 days	2–3 wk*	58–63	1½ yr	6–9 mo
Ferret†	4–15 days	In and out of heat throughout the spring	40–42	1 yr	5–7 mo

*Cats usually come in and out of heat from early spring to late summer. Variations can occur in different climates. In most cases, a female cat must be bred to produce an egg, which is why cats come into heat so frequently.
†Ferrets are prone to illness if not spayed. Unless you intend to breed your ferret, have her spayed.

GESTATION IN CATS AND DOGS

This chart can be used to estimate when to expect the litter. The chart is based on a 63-day gestation length. Variations occur, and gestation can range from 58 to 65 days. The first column gives the breeding date, and the second the birthing date (see next page).

QUEENING (BIRTHING OF KITTENS)

Cats usually have few problems giving birth to their kittens.

Signs of Queening
1. Two weeks before labor the nipples and breasts become prominent and pink.
2. One week before labor, the cat's activity decreases and she starts searching for a place to have her kittens. Begin to acquaint her with a box containing soft, clean cloth and located in a quiet area. Begin to take her temperature twice daily.
3. Twelve to twenty-four hours before labor, she'll show signs of restlessness. She'll experience frequent urination, and her rectal temperature will drop below 99°F.

Signs of Normal Labor
1. Open-mouthed breathing
2. Abdominal contractions
3. Lying on chest with hind legs extended
4. Crying and groaning

DELIVERY

The birth of the first kitten usually follows two to sixty minutes of hard labor. The second kitten usually follows in ten minutes to two

GESTATION IN CATS AND DOGS

Jan.	Mar.	Feb.	Apr.	Mar.	May	Apr.	June	May	July	June	Aug.
1	5	1	5	1	3	1	3	1	3	1	3
2	6	2	6	2	4	2	4	2	4	2	4
3	7	3	7	3	5	3	5	3	5	3	5
4	8	4	8	4	6	4	6	4	6	4	6
5	9	5	9	5	7	5	7	5	7	5	7
6	10	6	10	6	8	6	8	6	8	6	8
7	11	7	11	7	9	7	9	7	9	7	9
8	12	8	12	8	10	8	10	8	10	8	10
9	13	9	13	9	11	9	11	9	11	9	11
10	14	10	14	10	12	10	12	10	12	10	12
11	15	11	15	11	13	11	13	11	13	11	13
12	16	12	16	12	14	12	14	12	14	12	14
13	17	13	17	13	15	13	15	13	15	13	15
14	18	14	18	14	16	14	16	14	16	14	16
15	19	15	19	15	17	15	17	15	17	15	17
16	20	16	20	16	18	16	18	16	18	16	18
17	21	17	21	17	19	17	19	17	19	17	19
18	22	18	22	18	20	18	20	18	20	18	20
19	23	19	23	19	21	19	21	19	21	19	21
20	24	20	24	20	22	20	22	20	22	20	22
21	25	21	25	21	23	21	23	21	23	21	23
22	26	22	26	22	24	22	24	22	24	22	24
23	27	23	27	23	25	23	25	23	25	23	25
24	28	24	28	24	26	24	26	24	26	24	26
25	29	25	29	25	27	25	27	25	27	25	27
26	30	26	30	26	28	26	28	26	28	26	28
27	31			27	29	27	29	27	29	27	29
				28	30	28	30	28	30	28	30
				29	31			29	31	29	31
	Apr.		May		June		July		Aug.		Sept.
28	1	27	1	30	1	29	1	30	1	30	1
29	2	28	2	31	2	30	2	31	2		
30	3										
31	4										

July	Sept.	Aug.	Oct.	Sept.	Nov.	Oct.	Dec.	Nov.	Jan.	Dec.	Feb.
1	2	1	3	1	3	1	3	1	3	1	2
2	3	2	4	2	4	2	4	2	4	2	3
3	4	3	5	3	5	3	5	3	5	3	4
4	5	4	6	4	6	4	6	4	6	4	5
5	6	5	7	5	7	5	7	5	7	5	6
6	7	6	8	6	8	6	8	6	8	6	7
7	8	7	9	7	9	7	9	7	9	7	8
8	9	8	10	8	10	8	10	8	10	8	9
9	10	9	11	9	11	9	11	9	11	9	10
10	11	10	12	10	12	10	12	10	12	10	11
11	12	11	13	11	13	11	13	11	13	11	12
12	13	12	14	12	14	12	14	12	14	12	13
13	14	13	15	13	15	13	15	13	15	13	14
14	15	14	16	14	16	14	16	14	16	14	15
15	16	15	17	15	17	15	17	15	17	15	16
16	17	16	18	16	18	16	18	16	18	16	17
17	18	17	19	17	19	17	19	17	19	17	18
18	19	18	20	18	20	18	20	18	20	18	19
19	20	19	21	19	21	19	21	19	21	19	20
20	21	20	22	20	22	20	22	20	22	20	21
21	22	21	23	21	23	21	23	21	23	21	22
22	23	22	24	22	24	22	24	22	24	22	23
23	24	23	25	23	25	23	25	23	25	23	24
24	25	24	26	24	26	24	26	24	26	24	25
25	26	25	27	25	27	25	27	25	27	25	26
26	27	26	28	26	28	26	28	26	28	26	27
27	28	27	29	27	29	27	29	27	29	27	28
28	29	28	30	28	30	28	30	28	30		
29	30	29	31			29	31	29	31		
	Oct.		Nov.		Dec.		Jan.		Feb.		Mar.
30	1	30	1	29	1	30	1	30	1	28	1
31	2	31	2	30	2	31	2			29	2
										30	3
										31	4

hours. There may be a wait of up to twenty-four hours before the other kittens are born.

The mother cat will tear open the membrane covering each kitten and sever the cord. She will lick the kitten vigorously and may eat the afterbirth. *Note:* Remove the afterbirth before she eats it, if possible, as it may cause diarrhea.

BIRTHING PROBLEMS

1. If no kitten is produced after two hours of hard abdominal contractions, call your veterinarian.
2. If there is a time lag between kittens of greater than twelve hours, call your veterinarian.
3. If the mother cat does not tear open the membranes of her newly born kittens, follow the instructions given below in Whelping. The procedures are identical for puppies and kittens.
4. If the kittens are not yet nursing thirty to sixty minutes after birth, try to place them on the nipples. However, some mothers will not allow kittens to nurse until all have been delivered. Call your veterinarian if the situation persists.

Remember: See your veterinarian within twenty-four hours after the delivery to have both the mother cat and her kittens examined—if the queen hasn't hidden the kittens so well you can't find her nest.

WHELPING (BIRTHING OF PUPPIES)

Most dogs have no problem delivering their puppies if they are kept relatively alone and in a clean environment.

Signs of Whelping

1. Two weeks before labor, the mother dog's hair falls out around the nipples and the vulva becomes flaccid and swollen.

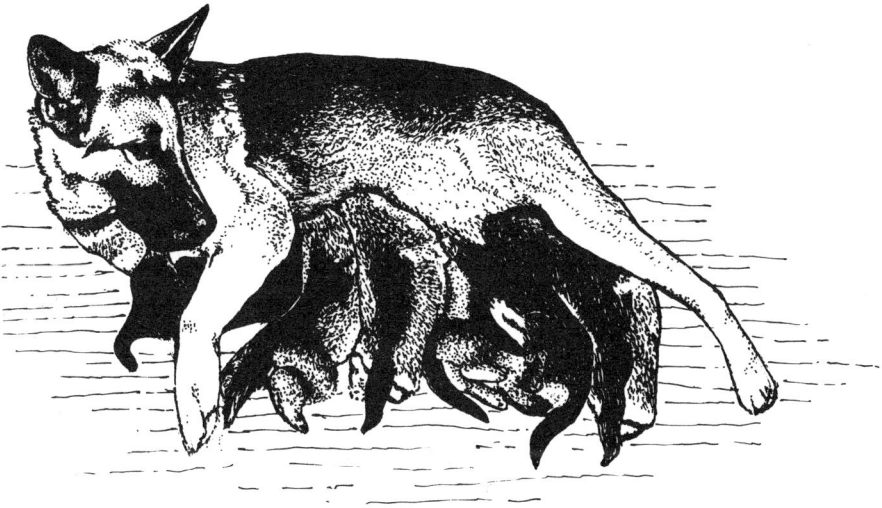

2. One week before labor, her appetite will often decrease. It is helpful to take your pet's temperature every twelve hours during the last week of pregnancy.
3. Twelve to twenty-four hours before labor, her rectal temperature will drop to below 99°F.
4. One to four hours before labor, she will become restless and her breathing rate will increase.

Signs of Normal Labor

1. Panting.
2. Abdominal spasms.
3. A brown-to-bloody discharge from the vulva.
4. The birth of the first puppy usually follows thirty to sixty minutes of labor.
5. There is usually a ten- to forty-five-minute interval between puppies.

DELIVERY

1. The mother licks the puppy as it is born. First-time mothers may not do this.
2. The puppy has been born. The cord is still attached to the placenta which is inside the mother. It will emerge very shortly. The sac covering the puppy has been removed by the mother.
3. The mother tears the cord with her teeth. Sometimes, especially if it is her first litter, she may cut the cord too short or tear the puppy's skin. If this happens, take the puppy to the veterinarian as soon as possible. Suturing this is very successful even if it looks disastrous.

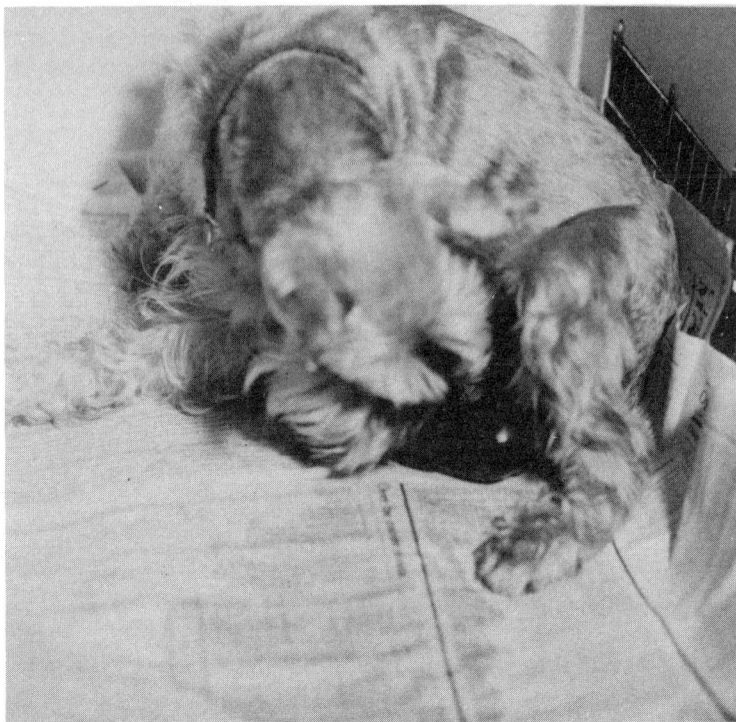

(1)

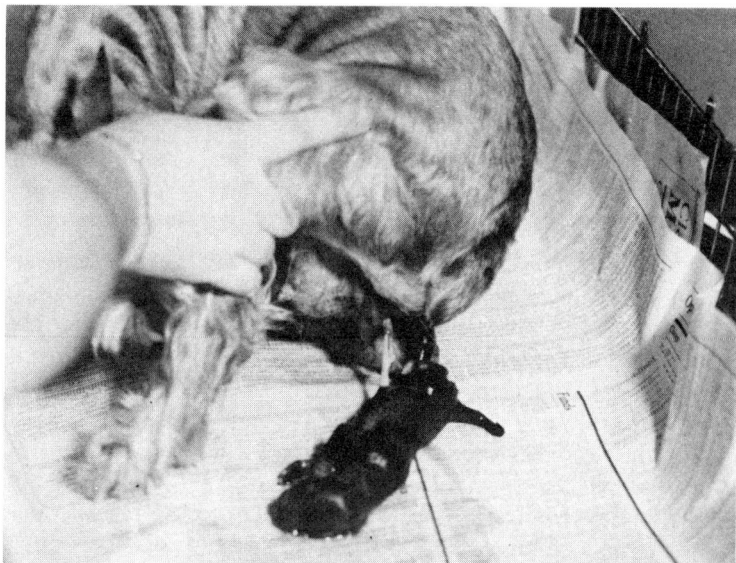

(2)

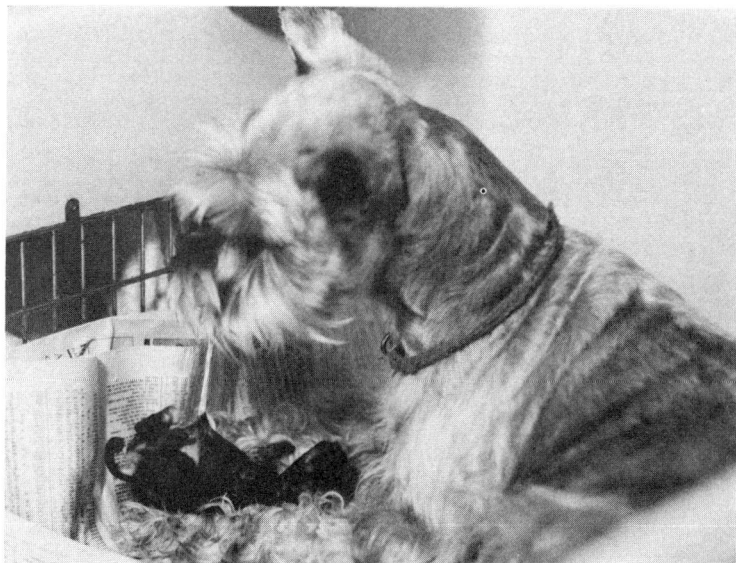

(3)

CARING FOR THE PUPPIES

First-time mothers often do not understand what is happening so they may not care for their puppies properly. If the mother does not break the sac or does not vigorously lick the puppy after it is born, you must follow the procedures outlined below.

1. Tear the sac with your fingers and remove the puppy. Clean any mucus or fluid out of its mouth.
2. With a warm towel, rub the puppy vigorously, but with little pressure. If the puppy does not start to breathe, carefully swing it between your legs in a rapid downward movement.
3. When the puppy is breathing, and the cord is still attached, cut the cord as directed below. It is normal for the breathing to look like gasps at first.
4. Continue rubbing the puppy to warm it and then place it near the mother's nipples. Be sure the puppies stay near her so they will be warmed by her body's heat. They should be nursing by the time she has finished giving birth, and by now the mother should be showing interest in her puppies.

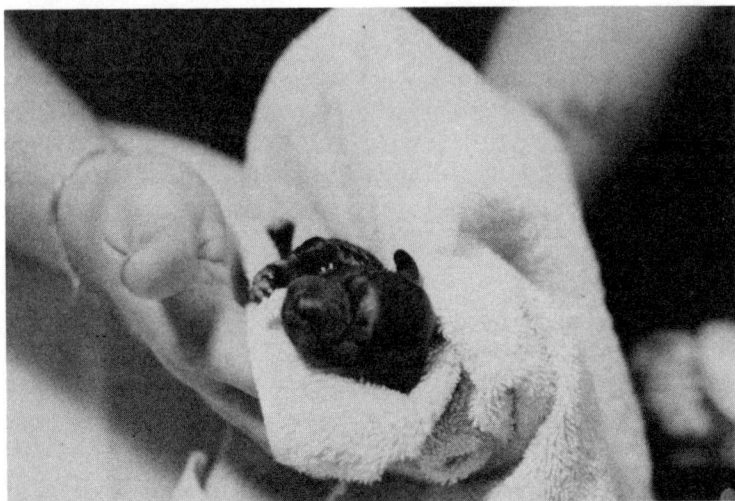

(1)

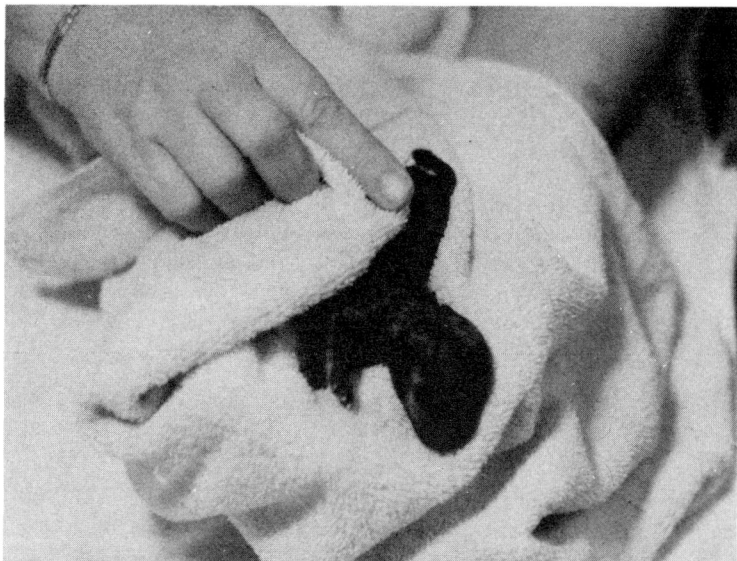

(2)

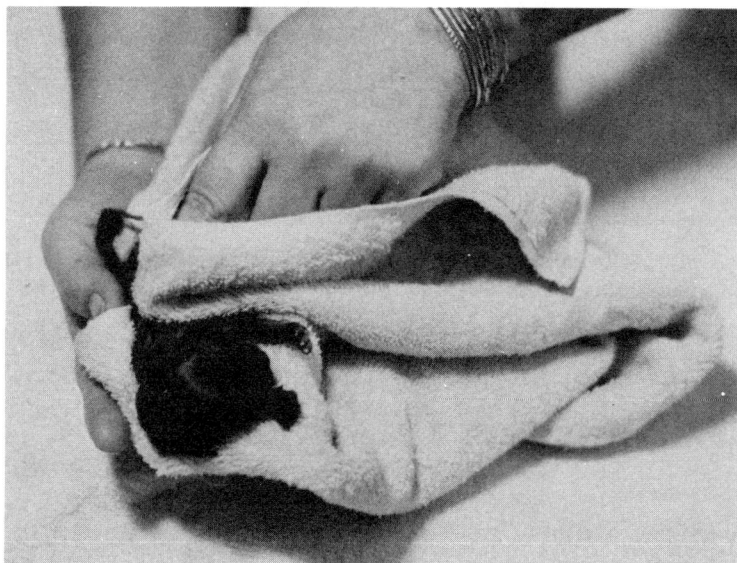

(3)

CUTTING THE CORD

If the mother has had puppies before, she will probably do this without any assistance for you. If not:

1. Use thread that has been boiled for twenty minutes.
2. Tie a square knot on the cord, one inch from the puppy.
3. Using sterile or recently washed scissors, cut the cord one-half inch beyond the tie.
4. Apply betadyne or iodine to the end of the cord.

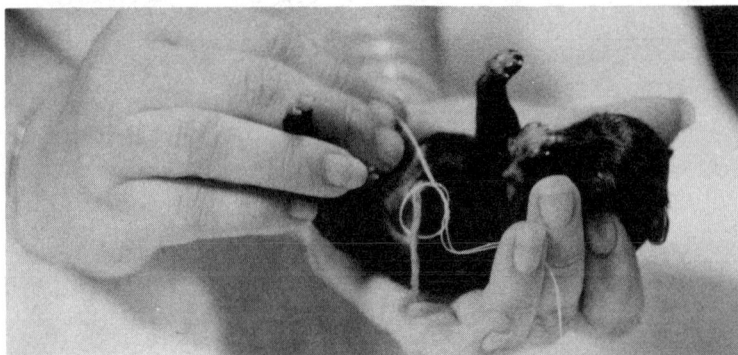

(1)

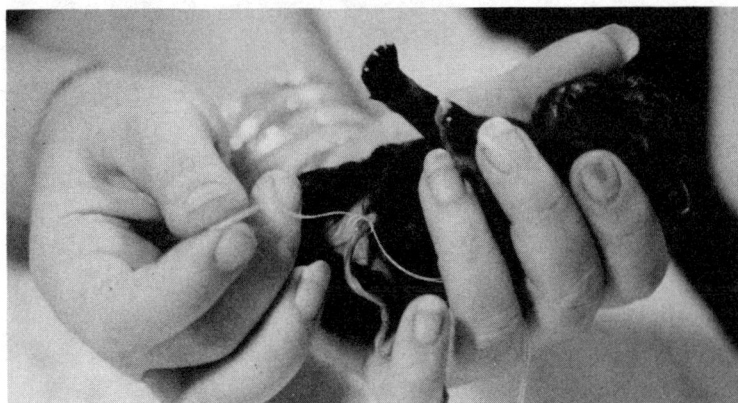

(2)

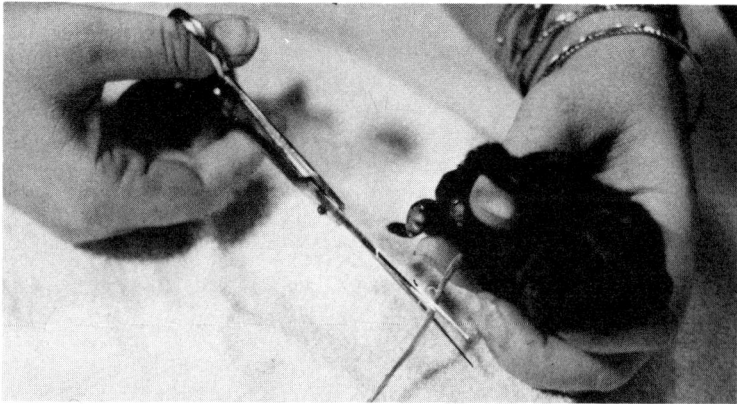

(3)

BIRTHING PROBLEMS

1. If there is a green discharge from the vulva before any puppies have been born, call your veterinarian immediately. This usually means the first puppy is dead.
2. If labor lasts longer than two hours without producing a puppy or if there is excessive straining for fifteen minutes without birth taking place, call your veterinarian immediately.
3. If the mother ignores her puppies at delivery, you must remove the birth sac from each puppy and tie the umbilical cord approximately one-half inch from the puppy's stomach. Cut the cord and apply tincture of iodine to its surface. Clean the mucus from the mouth, and massage the puppy gently but vigorously with warm towels until dry.
4. If there is more than one hour between deliveries, walk your pet and give her a little water.
5. If there is more than two hours between deliveries, call your veterinarian.
6. If a puppy is lodged partially out of the mother and is still, lubricate both the vulva and the puppy with K-Y jelly or another sterile lubricant. Gently pull the puppy out of the birth canal. If the puppy is lodged for more than ten minutes, it is probably dead and professional assistance is required immediately.

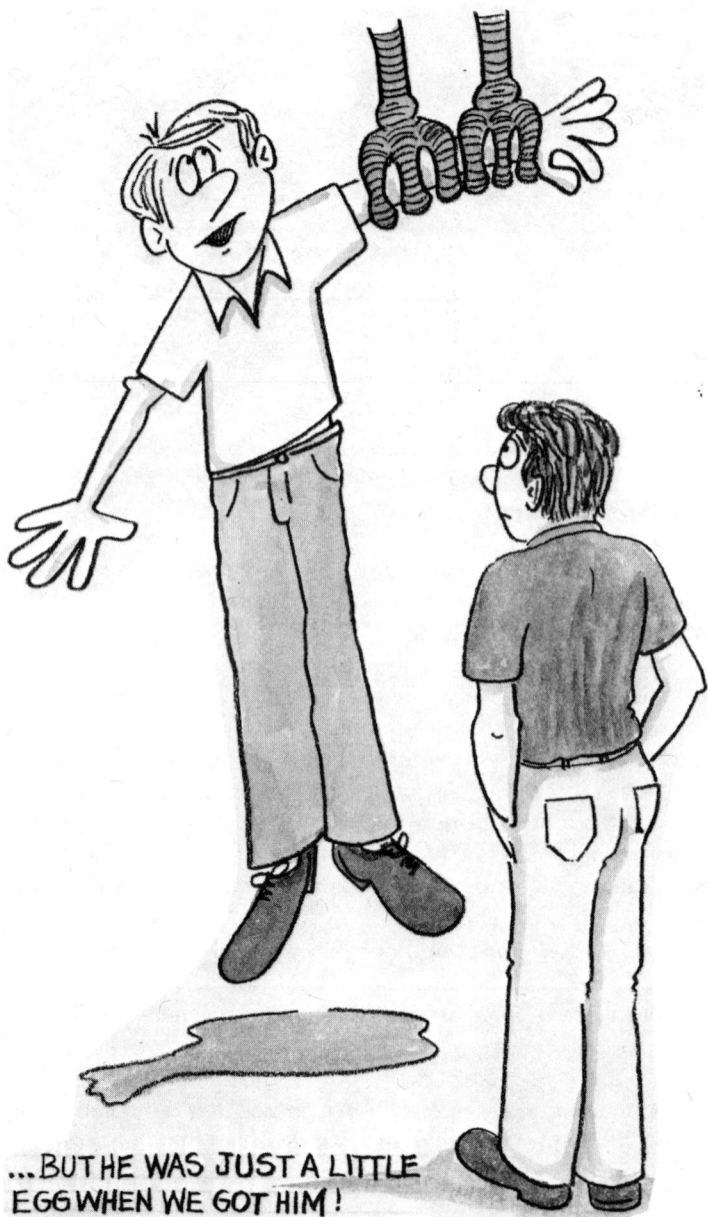

...BUT HE WAS JUST A LITTLE EGG WHEN WE GOT HIM!

CHAPTER FIVE
TENDING YOUR BIRD

GENERAL CARE AND DIET

The health of your bird will be ensured if you provide it the proper
housing and a stable environment; feed it a balanced diet of seeds,
fruits, and vegetables and supplement its diet with vitamins and
minerals; take it to the veterinarian for routine health examinations
two or three times a year; and learn to restrain and care for your
bird in emergency situations (see next page).

Symptoms of Illness

Birds have a great ability to mask illness and may be critically ill
before you realize the severity of the problem. At the first sign of
any illness, you should see your veterinarian. Any delay or improper
treatment can endanger the life of your pet. The signs include:

1. A discharge from the eyes
2. A change in the clarity or the color of the eyes
3. Closing the eyes
4. A discharge from the nostrils
5. Sneezing
6. A plugged nostril
7. An inability to manipulate or eat seeds
8. A reduction in, or loss of, appetite
9. Fluffed feathers
10. Inactivity
11. A break in normal routine
12. A change in, or stopping of, vocalization

13. Loss of weight
14. Loss of balance
15. An inability to perch
16. Crusty deposits on the nonfeathered portions of body
17. A change in the quality and or quantity of droppings
18. Open-mouth breathing
19. Bobbing or pumping of the tail
20. Bleeding

Note: Information specific to the health problems of birds is found in Chapter 2 under Bleeding, Egg Binding, Diarrhea, External and Internal Parasites, Poisoning, Seizures, Sneezing or Coughing, Trauma, and Vomiting.

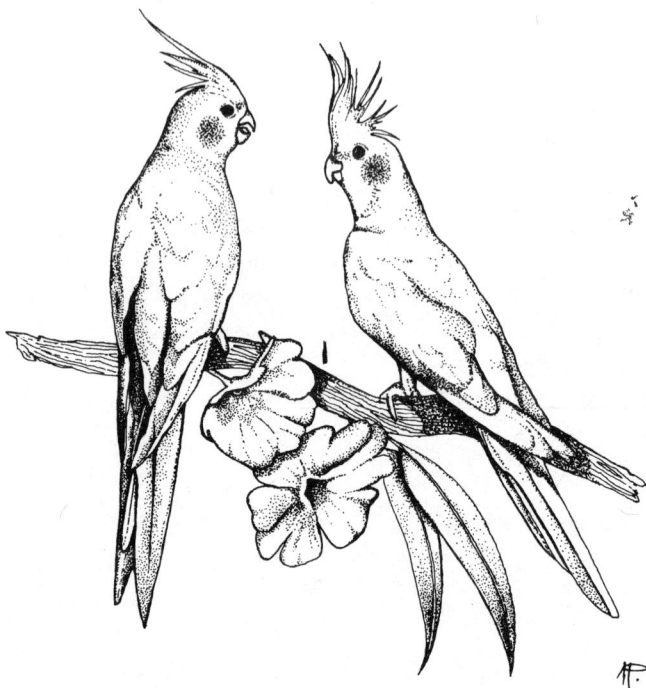

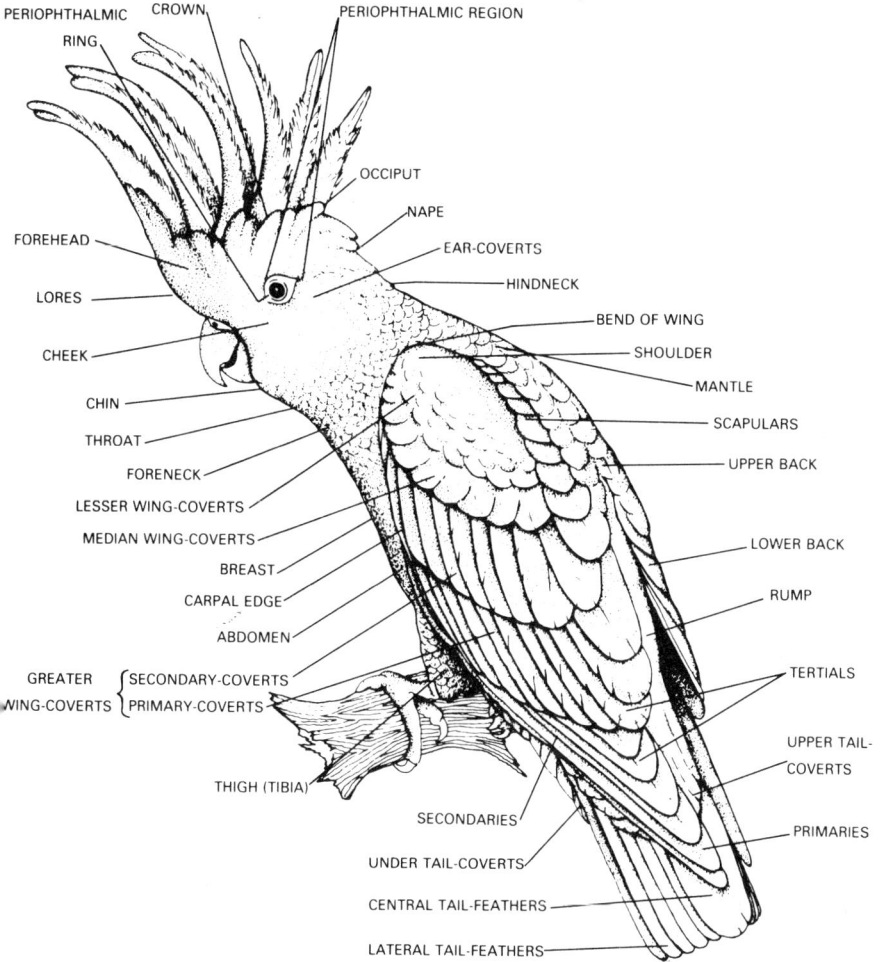

ANATOMY

PERIOPHTHALMIC
RING

CROWN

PERIOPHTHALMIC REGION

OCCIPUT

NAPE

FOREHEAD

EAR-COVERTS

LORES

HINDNECK

CHEEK

BEND OF WING

SHOULDER

CHIN

MANTLE

THROAT

SCAPULARS

FORENECK

UPPER BACK

LESSER WING-COVERTS

MEDIAN WING-COVERTS

LOWER BACK

BREAST

CARPAL EDGE

RUMP

ABDOMEN

GREATER
WING-COVERTS

SECONDARY-COVERTS

PRIMARY-COVERTS

TERTIALS

UPPER TAIL-
COVERTS

THIGH (TIBIA)

SECONDARIES

PRIMARIES

UNDER TAIL-COVERTS

CENTRAL TAIL-FEATHERS

LATERAL TAIL-FEATHERS

CHAPTER SIX

TENDING YOUR CAGED PET

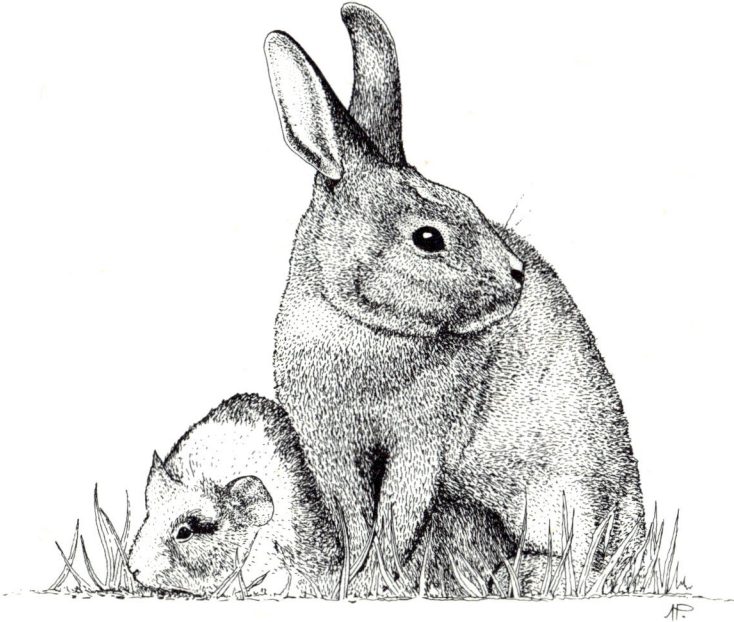

GENERAL CARE AND DIET

Many times we forget that the normal life span of our small caged
pets is only one to four years. (See the table below.) Having only
a brief time to enjoy them, we should be extra-solicitous to provide
them the proper diet, environment, and tender, loving care.

The proper diet includes water offered in a leak-proof bottle
feeder or in such a manner that it cannot be spilled or contaminated.
The proper food can be recommended for you by your veterinarian
or the store where you bought your pet. It is important that the food
be fresh and changed every day. Don't let it collect in the cage.

ANATOMY

Neck — Ear

Back —

Loin —

Flank — Face

Stifle —

Rump — Nose

Tail — Dewlap

Hock — Shoulder

Foot — Side

Claw — Elbow

Belly —

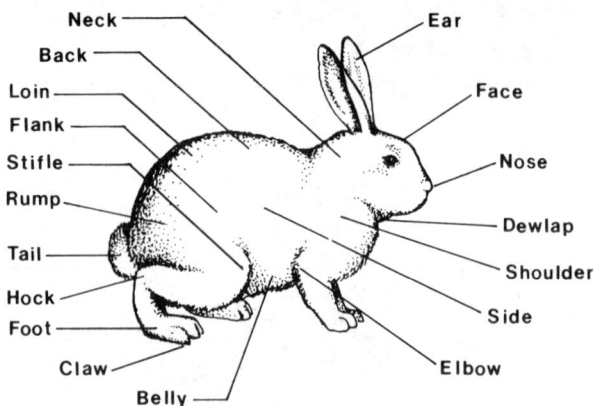

Note: Sometimes feeding greens can give your pet diarrhea. Feed these only in small amounts until you know your pet can eat them without any problem.

Note: Guinea pigs, unlike other pets, need vitamin C, so a diet rich in that vitamin, including fruits, vegetables, and a proper commercial mixture, must be fed on a regular basis.

The proper environment is assured if you provide your pet with a cage made specifically for that kind of animal. *Do not* close your pet up in a box; proper air circulation is important in order to prevent disease.

The cage should be placed in a warm location, away from drafts but with some indirect sunlight. It is very important that you keep it clean and dry. If bedding is required, you can use pine-wood shavings or a commercial bedding bought from your veterinarian or pet-supply store. Clean the cage at least twice a week.

Note: Information specific to the health problems of small caged pets is found in Chapter 2 under Diarrhea and Loss of Appetite.

FACTS OF LIFE FOR SMALL CAGED PETS

Animal	Life Span, yr	Body Temperature, °F	Length of Gestation, days	Litter Size	Eyes Open, days	Nursing Period	Eating Solid Food, days
Mouse	1–2	96.4–100	19–21	10–12	12–13	16–21 days	12–13
Hamster	1.6–2.5	97.2–99.5	16–18	6–8	15	20–24 days	7–9
Gerbil	4+	97.5–100.2	24–25	5	17–18	21–24 days	17–18
Rat	2–6	99.5–100.8	21–23	9–11	10–12	21 days	10–12
Guinea pig	6	100.4–102.2	65–72	3	At birth	14 days	5
Rabbit	6–7	102.2–103.2	31–32	8	10	6–8 weeks	21
Ferret	10–11	100–102	41–42	2–5	8–14	4–6 weeks	21

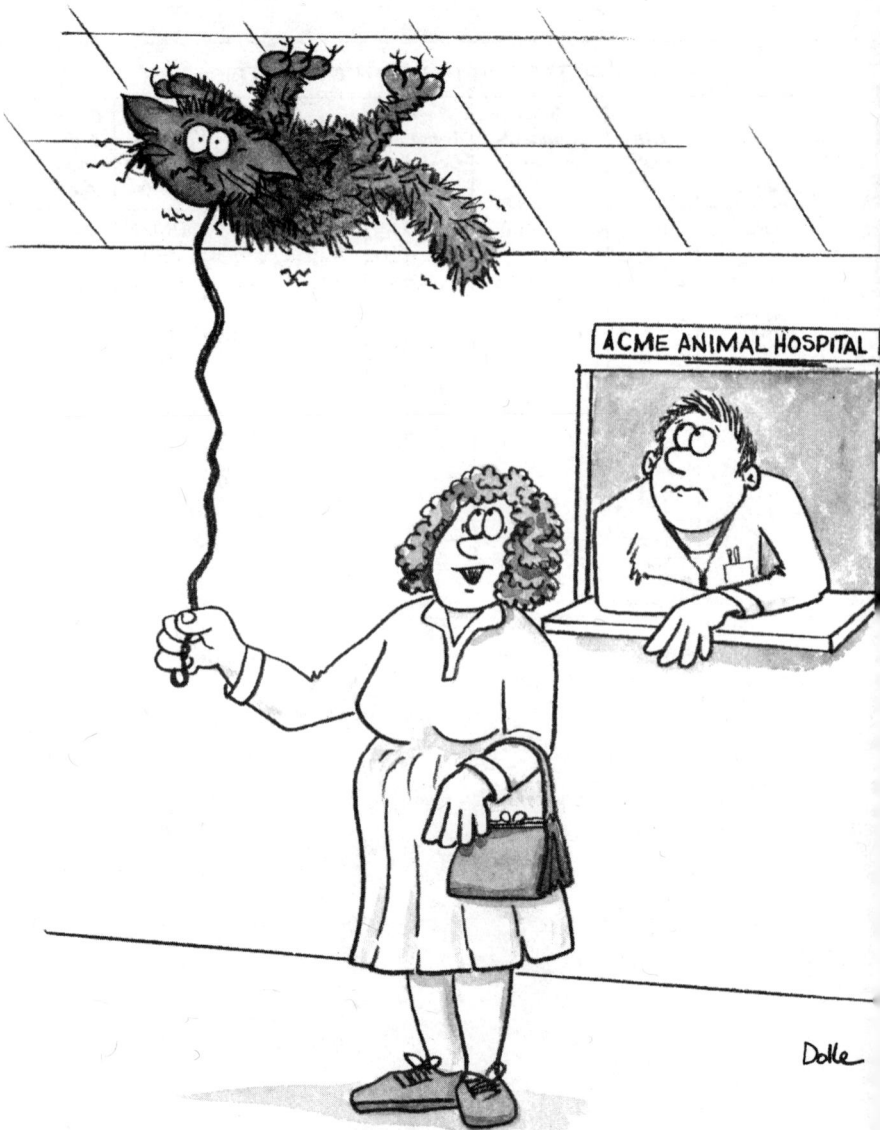

GEE DOC, MAYBE NEXT TIME YOU
SHOULD SPELL VACCINATION!

CHAPTER SEVEN

TENDING YOUR CAT OR DOG

GENERAL CARE AND DIET

Providing a good environment for your pet is important to his or her health. Food and water should be made available to pets at regular times, and shelter from dampness and cold should be provided for outdoor pets. Dogs that are kept indoors should be walked regularly. Cat litter boxes should be kept clean and fresh. Remember to give your pet loving attention when you have been away for long periods of time. A safe, caring environment will help your dog or cat thrive.

Choosing a diet for your dog or cat is an important part of preventive health care. Any food chosen should contain the pet's minimum daily requirements for nutrients and energy in a form usable by the dog or cat and acceptable to him or her. Commercial pet foods are more likely to meet these standards than even the most carefully prepared homemade pet meals. Based on his or her knowledge of your pet, your veterinarian can help you choose an acceptable brand of dry, soft-moist, or canned dog or cat food. Keep in mind that the best commercial pet foods have been formulated to meet the specific needs of cats or dogs, but not both, since there are significant differences in their needs.

The proper diet for your pet depends upon several other factors, including the animal's age, state of health, size, and activity level. Kittens and puppies need more nutrients than cats and dogs, and commercial kitten and puppy foods can provide those nutrients. Because of reduced activity, older cats and dogs require fewer calories per pound of body weight, and some older pets may need special diets.

During gestation and lactation, females require well-balanced diets beyond the maintenance diets that normally meet the needs of adult cats and dogs. Your veterinarian can recommend a special diet designed to provide the additional nutrients and higher levels of energy needed for successful birthing and nursing of kittens or puppies.

On a per-pound basis, smaller dogs require more energy than larger ones. Ranch dogs generally require more energy than city-dwelling house pets. Most cats and some dogs adjust well to self-feeding from a dish of dry food, but others are gluttons whose food intake must be regulated by their owners in order to prevent obesity.

FACTS OF LIFE FOR CATS AND DOGS

	Cat	Dog
Life span (years)	13–17	9–17
Body temperature (°F)	100.5–102.5	100.5–102.5
Length of gestation (days)	58–64	58–63
Litter size	3–5	4–8
Eyes open (days)	8–10	10–16
Nursing period (weeks)	6–8	6–8
Eating solid food (days)	28	21–28

VACCINATION SCHEDULES

Your new puppy or kitten or your unvaccinated adult cat or dog is susceptible to many infections. During their first few weeks of life, baby animals receive immunity from their mothers. When this temporary immunity wears off, vaccination is a safe and effective way to provide your pet with continued protection from many diseases. The following timetables represent acceptable vaccination programs for your cat or dog. Since variations may occur throughout the United States and abroad, according to regional outbreaks of disease, you should consult your veterinarian concerning vaccinations for your pet.

ANATOMY OF CAT

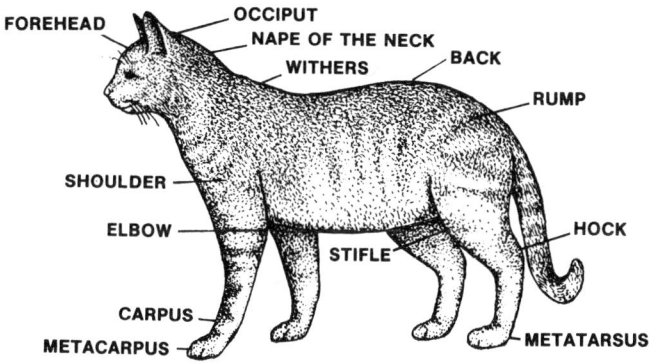

FOREHEAD
OCCIPUT
NAPE OF THE NECK
WITHERS
BACK
RUMP
SHOULDER
ELBOW
HOCK
STIFLE
CARPUS
METACARPUS
METATARSUS

ANATOMY OF DOG

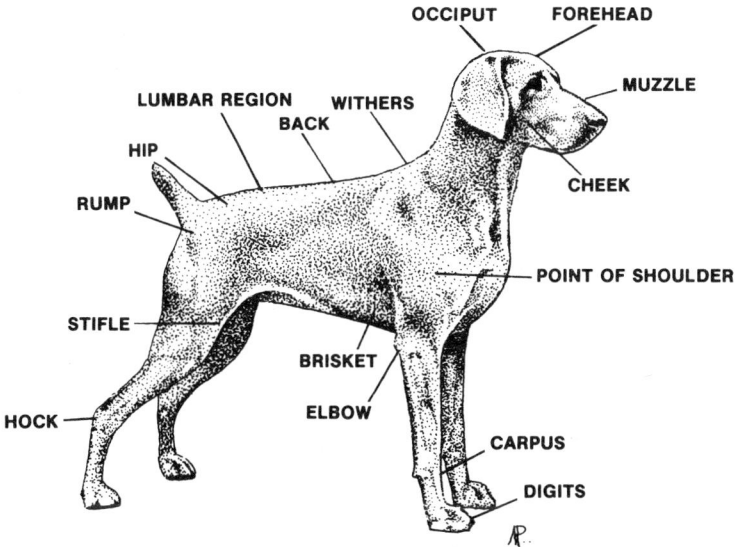

OCCIPUT
FOREHEAD
MUZZLE
LUMBAR REGION
WITHERS
BACK
HIP
CHEEK
RUMP
STIFLE
POINT OF SHOULDER
BRISKET
ELBOW
HOCK
CARPUS
DIGITS

TIMETABLE FOR CATS	
Vaccine*	**Age in weeks**
Rabies	16
Panleukopenia (fe-line distemper)	6–8, 9, 12
Viral rhinotracheitis	6–8, 9, 12
Calicivirus	6–8, 9, 12
Pneumonitis	6–8, 9, 12
Leukemia†	9, 12, 24

*Annual boosters are required on all cats for all the diseases listed. Variation in the frequency of vaccination can occur in show cats, cats in catteries, and cats living in areas where outbreaks of disease occur.
†A very effective vaccine is now available. Initially, all cats should have three vaccinations, spaced as recommended by your veterinarian.

TIMETABLE FOR DOGS	
Vaccine*	**Age in weeks**
Rabies	16
Distemper	6, 9, 12, 15
Measles	6
Hepatitis	9, 12, 15
Leptospirosis	9, 12, 15
Parainfluenza	9, 12, 15
Parvovirus†	6, 9, 12, 15

*Annual boosters are necessary on all the diseases listed except measles.
†Show dogs, working dogs, or any dog exposed to disease might need this vaccine every six months.

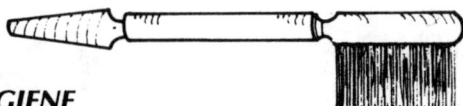

ORAL HYGIENE

Your pet's mouth should be examined by your veterinarian periodically. The veterinarian may recommend professional cleaning of your pet's teeth. Once the plaque has been removed, you should brush your pet's teeth one or two times a week to help prevent it from rebuilding.

If you begin brushing your pet's teeth when he or she is a puppy or kitten, your pet will usually accept the procedure without any protest and you will be helping your pet by practicing good preventive health care.

Good oral hygiene will help reduce tooth-plaque buildup and

decrease risk of gum disease, infection, and abscess, which could lead to systemic infections, pain, and suffering.

Note: There are many causes of bad breath in animals, including poor nutrition, gum disease, plaque, infection, and kidney failure.

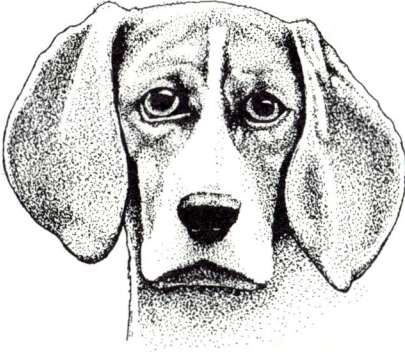

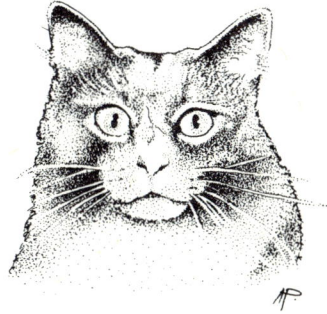

CHAPTER EIGHT

TENDING WILD BABY ANIMALS AND BIRDS

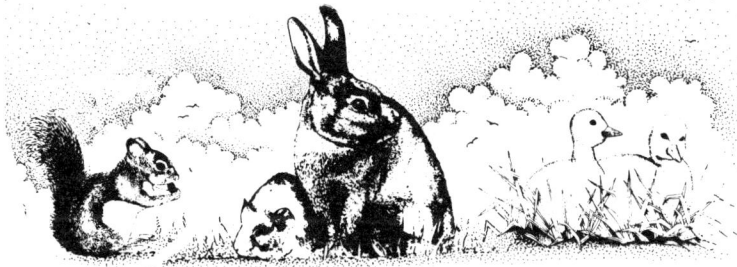

If a small wild animal or a bird has been injured, call your veterinarian or the local Audobon Society for assistance. Always wear gloves and thoroughly wash your hands after handling these orphans. *Do not handle raccoons, skunks, foxes, bats, ground squirrels* (in the western states), *or prairie dogs* because they can carry deadly diseases. Remember, any injured animal should be returned to the wild when it is well enough to care for itself because that's where it will be happiest.

Like any domestic animal, a wild animal needs the proper environment and diet in order to thrive. All baby animals and birds must be kept warm. (Three methods of ensuring a warm environment are presented under Trauma in Chapter 2.) Always be sure the cage is sufficiently secure so that the orphan cannot escape and no other animals can reach it. Keep the cage in a quiet place away from drafts.

The proper diet will vary according to the kind of animal:

Squirrels and mice: Mix one egg yolk and one-half cup milk (evaporated preferred); either one tablespoon honey, Veterinarian's High-Energy Formula, or Karo syrup; a pinch of salt. Blend well and heat to almost a boil. Let mixture cool to room temperature. With an eyedropper feed the mixture to the animal every one to three hours. (Feed young and weak animals more often.) This mixture will last five days in the refrigerator. When the orphan is two to three weeks of age, add breakfast cereal, nuts, and fruit to its diet.

Rabbits: Feed the same as above but add dry breakfast cereal and leafy green vegetables when the animal is older.

Opossum: Feed the same as above but mix canned dog food with the formula when the animal is older.

Quail, chickens, and ducklings: Mix one-half cup dry bread crumbs with one hard-boiled egg yolk and enough milk to make crumbly. Feed this in tiny pellets. As the bird gets older, add chick starter and leafy green vegetables.

Song birds: Gently place small pellets made of a canned dog food dipped in formula (egg yolk and one-half cup milk, one tablespoon honey or Veterinarians's High-Energy Formula, one-fourth teaspoon salt) into the bird's mouth every two to three hours.

The formulas given above will contain enough water to supply the needs of baby mammals. Birds, however, will require more water. After the baby bird has finished each feeding, slowly offer water with a dropper.

Note: Baby animals must be stimulated to urinate and defecate. Gently rub the anus with a warm, wet cloth of a very soft material.

Should the animal give any evidence of diarrhea or loss of appetite, see the discussions of those two disorders in Chapter 2.

OLD WIVES' TALES

Don't Believe That . . .

Brewer's yeast fed to your pet will kill fleas.

Cats will suffocate a baby by inhaling through the nostrils of the sleeping infant.

Burnt motor oil applied to your dog's skin will cure red mange.

Saliva from a dog's mouth is all that is needed to heal a wound.

A rubber band applied to a dog's tail is good for tail docking.

Spiderwebs are good for stopping a surface wound from bleeding.

A dog will become insane unless she has a litter of puppies before being spayed.

A dry nose means your pet has a fever.

Dewclaws on the back feet of dogs make them immune to snake bites.

You can worm a dog with a copper penny.

Neutering a pet automatically makes it gain weight.

You can't teach an old dog new tricks.

A drop of tincture of iodine in the food prevents heartworms.

Slitting a bird's tongue helps it talk better. (Disfiguration and death from bleeding may result.)

Bread, candy, or potatoes give your pet worms.

Rolling an unboiled egg over your pet will cure a fever.

APPENDIX B

CONVERTING A DOG'S AGE INTO HUMAN YEARS

Dog's Age	Equivalent Human Age, yr
6 mo	10
8 mo	13
10 mo	14
12 mo	15
18 mo	20
2 yr	24
4 yr	32
6 yr	40
8 yr	48
10 yr	56
12 yr	64
14 yr	72
16 yr	80
18 yr	88
20 yr	96
21 yr	100

COMMON VETERINARY TERMS

Abdomen—The portion of the body between the chest and the hind legs which contains the stomach, intestines, liver, kidneys, pancreas, and other organs.

Abscess—A localized accumulation of pus.

Acute—Having a short and severe course or duration.

Anal sacs—Two saclike structures located just under the skin on either side of the anus.

Anemia—A low number of red cells in the blood.

Antibiotic—A substance that slows or destroys the growth of microorganisms.

Antibody—A protein produced by the body's immune system to help prevent infection.

Antiseptic—A substance which kills bacteria and is used externally.

Arthritis—Inflammation of any joint.

Bacteria—A microscopic organism which may cause disease.

Betadyne—An iodine-based antiseptic.

Cancer (malignant)—A cancer which spreads to surrounding tissues.

Caesarean section—A surgical procedure to remove baby animals from the mother's uterus when she is unable to deliver them naturally.

Castration—A surgical procedure to remove the testicles of a male animal so he cannot breed.

Cere—A waxy, often brightly colored, fleshy area at the base of the beak of birds such as parrots, hawks, and eagles; includes the nostrils.

Chronic—A term used to describe an illness or disease which has been continuing for an extended period of time or which has been recurring.

Cloaca—In birds, an opening under the base of the tail feathers for the elimination of urine and feces.

Coccidia—A one-celled protozoan parasite of the intestinal tract that can cause loss of appetite, diarrhea, and blood in stools.

Compound fracture—A break in a bone in which a portion of the bone has penetrated through the skin, or a break which has an open wound from the skin down to the bone.

Congenital—Present at the time of birth.

Conjunctivitis—Inflammation of the thin membrane which lines the inside of the eyelids and extends down over the white portion of the eyeball.

Coonhound paralysis—A viral disease of dogs carried by raccoons and possibly other wild animals; results in death if not treated.

Cortisone—A drug which reduces inflammation.

Cystitis—Inflammation of the urinary bladder.

Demodectic mange (red mange)—A noncontagious skin condition of dogs characterized by hair loss, reddening of the skin, and generalized inflammation and infection; caused by a small mite that lives in the skin and hair follicles.

Diabetes mellitus—High levels of glucose (sugar) in the blood and urine due to a lack of insulin production or utilization; usually causes weight loss and increased drinking of water.

Distemper, canine—A contagious viral disease that may have a variety of symptoms, including a discharge from the nose and eyes, pneumonia, diarrhea, muscle twitching or jerking, and, in severe cases, seizures.

Distemper, feline—A severe, contagious viral disease of cats which causes loss of appetite, depression, vomiting, diarrhea, and high mortality, especially in young kittens.

Eclampsia (Milk Fever)—Low blood levels of calcium in female animals that are nursing their young. Signs include restlessness, muscle twitching, collapse, and convulsions and may end in death if not treated properly.

Edema—Excessive fluid buildup in body tissues.

Enteritis—Inflammation of the intestine; causes include bacteria, viruses, and spoiled food.

Epilepsy—A disturbance of normal brain function which causes a partial or complete loss of consciousness, periods of altered behavior, or convulsions.

Eyelid, third—The transparent tissue attached to the inner side or lower lid of the eye of mammals; protects the eye and keeps it moist.

Fecal—Referring to stools (feces or excrement).

Feline leukemia—A usually fatal, contagious viral disease of cats which affects many organs of the body and often produces anemia, infections, abscesses, depression, cancer, and a chronic immunodeficiency. Treatment is often of no help. There is now a vaccine available through your veterinarian to prevent this disease.

Frostbite—An injury to a portion of the body, usually the extremities or exposed parts, resulting from prolonged exposure to frigid temperatures.

Fungus—A simple plant that can cause disease in the skin or any organ. Many are not harmful and are found in the environment.

Gangrene—The decay or destruction of soft body tissue due to disease or a loss of blood supply to a specific part of the body.

Gastritis—An inflammation of the lining of the stomach.

Granulation—The process of wound healing characterized by the formation of rough, reddish granules on the surface of the wound.

Hairball—Hair that is swallowed during grooming or licking and collects in the digestive tract. It can cause vomiting, constipation, or an intestinal blockage.

Heartworms—A parasite spread by mosquitoes to dogs (rarely cats) which lives in the heart.

Hematoma—A swelling due to a collection of blood under the skin. It is often seen as a swollen, painful ear in dogs and cats.

Hemorrhage—Bleeding from some part of the body.

Hepatitis—Inflammation of the liver due to a variety of causes ranging from infection to poison.

Hernia—A weak spot or tear in the muscle wall of a body cavity. Protrusion of the organs is common.

Hip dysplasia—An hereditary condition usually affecting the hips of large breeds; causes lameness, slowness to rise, or pain. It is diagnosed by x-ray.

Hookworms—A sometimes fatal intestinal parasite of the digestive tract characterized by weight loss, dull coat, anemia, and blood in the stool.

Hot spot—A rapidly occurring, localized area of redness, tenderness, itching, bleeding, or infection caused by a variety of conditions.

Inflammation—The body's response to infection or injury; characterized by swelling, redness, pain, irritation, or loss of function.

Intramuscular (IM) injection—An injection into the muscle.

Intravenous (IV) injection—An injection into the vein.

Jugular vein—The large vein on either side of an animal's neck. It is used by your veterinarian to obtain blood samples.

Kaopectate—An antidiarrheal drug available in pharmacies.

Leptospirosis—A bacterial disease which often causes kidney and liver failure and affects people and animals. There is a vaccination available for it.

Mange—See Demodectic mange, Scabies.

Mastitis—An inflammation or infection of the breasts characterized by hot, painful breasts or discolored milk. Remove the young, if nursing, and take the mother for treatment as soon as possible.

Microfilaria—The microscopic young of nematodes; in heartworm disease, they are seen in the blood.

Mites—Small parasites that chew or suck blood; can be found in the ears, skin, or feathers and cause infection, mange, hair loss, or skin irritation.

Necrotic—Dead or dying, as in necrotic tissue caused by infection, inflammation, or loss of blood supply.

Neuter—To castrate or spay pets; usually refers to males.

Ovariohysterectomy—A surgical procedure in the female which removes the ovaries and uterus; "spay" is the common term.

Panleukopenia—A very contagious viral disease in cats characterized by vomiting, diarrhea, depression, and death. Commonly called "feline distemper." Your veterinarian has a vaccine to prevent this.

Parasite—An organism living in or on another animal. It depends on the animal to survive and can cause poor health or even death in its host.

Parvovirus—A highly contagious, often fatal, viral disease in dogs characterized by vomiting and bloody diarrhea. Young dogs (less than two years old) are most susceptible. There is a vaccine for this.

Peritonitis—Inflammation of the abdominal cavity caused by infection or a foreign substance.

Placenta (afterbirth)—The membrane or covering of the fetus in the uterus.

Pneumonia—A disease in the lungs caused by bacteria, viruses, cancer, allergic reactions, or parasites. It is characterized by coughing, difficulty in breathing, fever, and loss of appetite.

Prolapsed eyeball—A traumatic condition in which the eye pops out of its socket.

Protozoa—A one-celled parasite of the gastrointestinal tract.

Pyometra—Pus in the uterus.

Queen—A fertile female cat.

Queening—Giving birth in cats.

Rabies—A contagious viral disease of the nervous system of mammals transmitted through saliva. It is a fatal disease in humans, dogs, and cats. There is a vaccination for this disease.

Ringworm—A contagious skin disease caused by a fungus. It may be characterized by itching and round, hairless areas.

Roundworm—A species of worm that lives as a parasite in the intestine. Its name is derived from its shape.

Scabies (sarcoptic mange)—A contagious skin disease caused by a mite (*Sarcoptes*) which burrows under the skin; severe itching is seen with this disease.

Shock—Ineffective circulation caused by injury, bleeding, infection, or a heart disturbance. Decreased blood pressure, rapid pulse, paleness, and death may result.

Spay—To remove the ovaries and uterus from a female animal, making her no longer fertile.

Stool—Fecal matter evacuated by a bowel movement.

Stress—Mental or physical tension or strain caused by pressure or any nonroutine activity.

Subcutaneous injection—An injection beneath the skin.

Suture—To join together the edges of a wound or incision by stitching; also, the material used to surgically close a wound or laceration.

Tapeworm—A species of worm living in the intestine.

Ticks—Wingless, blood-sucking, external parasites larger than, but related to, mites; some types can transmit disease and cause paralysis.

Trauma—Bodily injury or wounding.

Tumor—A mass of new tissue that grows independent of its surrounding structure and has no normal function.

Urinary calculi—An abnormal accumulation of mineral salts in any part of the urinary tract.

Vagina—In the female the canal extending from the vulva to the cervix of the uterus.

Virus—An infectious organism capable of reproducing only in living cells and too small to be seen with a microscope.

Vulva—The opening of the external genital organs of the female; the entrance to the vagina.

Whelping—Giving birth in dogs.

Whipworm—A dangerous intestinal parasite which has a whiplike front portion and is about two inches long.

EQUIVALENT WEIGHTS AND MEASURES

WEIGHT

1 gram (g) = 0.035 ounce (oz)
1 kilogram (kg) = 2.2 pound (lb) = 1000 g
1 milligram (mg) = 1/1000 g = 0.001 g
1 microgram (μg) = 1/1,000,000 g = 0.000001 g
1 oz = 28.5 g
1 lb = 454.0 gm = 0.45 kg

VOLUME

1 milliliter (mL) = 1/1,000 liter (L) = 1 cubic centimeter (cc)
1 L = 1000 mL = 1.1 quarts (qt)
1 fluid ounce (fl oz) = 30 mL = 2 tablespoons (tbsp)
1 qt = 0.95 L = 946.0 mL
1 teaspoon (tsp) = 5 mL = 60 drops (approximately)
1 tbsp = 14 mL = 3 tsp

LENGTH

1 centimeter (cm) = 0.39 inch (in)
1 meter (m) = 39.4 in = 1000 millimeters (mm) = 100 cm
1 kilometer (km) = 0.62 mile (mi) = 1000 m
1 mm = 0.039 in = 1/1,000 m
1 in = 2.54 cm
1 foot (ft) = 30.48 cm

LENGTH (con't)

1 yard (yd) = 0.91 m
1 mi = 1.6 km

TEMPERATURE

To convert Fahrenheit to Celsius, subtract 32 and multiply by 5/9.
To convert Celsius to Fahrenheit, multiply by 9/5 and add 32.

PET FIRST-AID INFORMATION

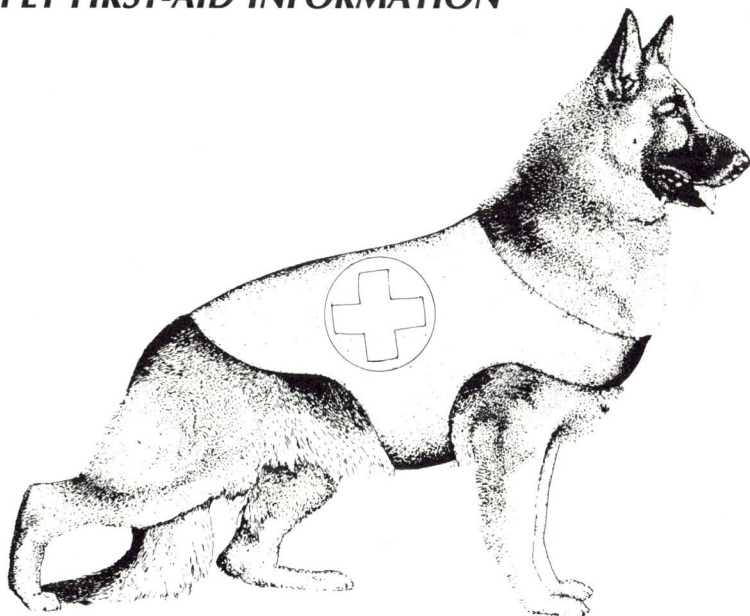

For information concerning first-aid products, pet-safety products, or questions pertaining to procedures for first aid write:

PET FIRST AID
P. O. BOX 14992
ORLANDO, FL 32857

Include:

1. Your name and address
2. Stamped self-addressed envelope
3. Type and number of pet(s)
4. Questions about pet first aid
5. Products you are interested in

INDEX

Catalog

If you are interested in a list of fine Paperback
books, covering a wide range of subjects
and interests, send your name and address,
requesting your free catalog, to:

McGraw-Hill Paperbacks
1221 Avenue of Americas
New York, N.Y. 10020